Contents

Preface

Nursing historically can lay claim to case management since the days of providing service coordination in public health during the turn of the century. Today, nurses play an integral role in all arenas of health care delivery, with care coordination as the hallmark of their practice. Through the efforts of nurse case managers, clients and families are assessed and an appropriate plan of care is developed to provide for essential services. Such efforts have shown that cost-effective care can be provided in an atmosphere of patient advocacy.

Since the publication of *Nursing Case Management* by the American Nurses Association (1988), case management by nurses has grown and taken on new forms. This new publication is intended to be a guide for continued development and expansion of case management practice. Use the models presented herein as starting points to expand upon individual or agency practice, and to recommit to a spirit of client advocacy. Nursing case management can be a solution to many of today's health care problems.

LINDA R. CRONENWETT, Ph.D., R.N., F.A.A.N.
Chairperson, ANA Congress of Nursing Practice

Introduction

Monumental changes in the provision of health care have occurred during the past several years. Advances in technology, restructuring of payment strategies for health care, reduced lengths of hospital stay, an aging population, increasing numbers of chronically ill clients, and alternative sites for care are some of the factors contributing to dramatic changes within the health care system.

Although many of these changes have been beneficial, there is persistent dissatisfaction with the nation's health care delivery system. Clients and other consumers are overwhelmed by limited access to care, escalating costs, the complexity of the system, and fragmentation of care. Providers are equally overwhelmed by the sharp rise in the acuity and complexity of patient care problems. Health care institutions are pressured by the demands of multiple constituencies who are perceived to have mutually exclusive needs. Simultaneously, payers must respond to their constituencies' demands for quality care at a lower cost, as employers and government agencies react to the escalating portions of their dollars that are spent on health care costs.

To further complicate the picture of health care today, services often are provided in several care settings and by multiple providers, contributing to the fragmentation of care. This is especially true for the chronically ill and the elderly. Yet these are client populations with complex problems, demanding careful coordination and skillful management.

The provision of outcome-oriented, cost-effective health care is no longer a goal — it is a mandate. To accomplish this mandate, the relationship between the costs of care, the desired outcomes of care, and the processes involved in providing care must be reexamined. The current frustrations stem, in part, from a disequilibrium of these three factors. The costs, processes, and outcomes of care are interrelated and reciprocal — changes in one aspect (such as reductions in cost) can have a significant effect on the others. Health care delivery must be restructured and refocused to attain an effective balance between costs, desired outcomes, and processes for delivery of care.

Case management* has emerged as a strategy to focus on the problems and needs of clients, as well as the families and friends who support their problems and needs, while maintaining a balance between outcome, cost, and process. The overall purpose of case management is to advocate for the patient through coordination of care, which reduces fragmentation and, ultimately, cost. Nurses have played a vital role in case management since its inception, and they currently function in this role in multiple health care arenas. Public health nurses have a long history as case managers. Similarly, psychiatric-mental health nurses have provided case management services for years. When some insurance companies introduced case management programs a number of years ago as a means of controlling costs while maintaining client outcomes and satisfaction, nurses were (and continue to be) employed in case management roles. Within the past few years, nurses in inpatient settings (including acute care) have incorporated the principles and techniques of case management into their practice, and are developing new models of nursing case management. Case management maximizes the effective utilization of the broad skills and knowledge base nurses bring to their practice. Nurses practicing as case managers are positioned as links between the quality and cost-effective aspects of care.

**Case management* should not be confused with *managed care*, another relatively recent development in health care delivery. Case management refers to patient-focused strategies to coordinate care. Managed care refers to strategies employed by purchasers of health services to influence aggregate utilization levels of various types of services in order to maintain quality and control costs. Managed care arrangements, such as health maintenance organizations (HMOs) and preferred provider organizations (PPOs), do not emphasize individual, client-level care coordination, as does case management. [It should be noted, however, that managed care programs which often do not fit this description are emerging.]

The Concept of Case Management

Case management is a paradoxically simple yet complex concept. The fundamental focus of case management is to integrate, coordinate, and advocate for individuals, families, and groups requiring extensive services. The ultimate goal is to achieve planned care outcomes by brokering services across the health care continuum. Although case management may be directed toward other goals, and although the primary purpose for instituting a case management system may vary among programs, coordination of care is the basic component of all models and modalities of case management. The term "case management" is generic, and modifiers are beginning to emerge to differentiate the various case management models.

Case management exists within many contexts and settings, including:

- insurance-based programs,
- employer-based programs,
- workers' compensation programs,
- social services programs,
- independent practice,
- medical practice,
- nursing practice,
- public health nursing and Visiting Nurse Association practices,
- maternal-child health settings, and
- mental health settings.

Case management can simultaneously be described as a system, a role, a technology, a process, and a service.

As a *system*, case management has many elements:

- Assessment and problem identification.
- Planning.
- Procurement, delivery, and coordination of services.
- Monitoring to assure that the multiple service needs of the client are met.

Case management also can be viewed as a clinical system that "focuses on the achievement of patient outcomes within effective and appropriate time frames and resources. Case management focuses on the entire episode of illness, crossing all settings in which the patient receives care" (Zander, 1990).

As a *role*, case management provides clients with a practitioner who actively coordinates their care. Within this role, the case manager is vested with the authority and accountability required to negotiate with multiple providers and obtain diverse services. The case manager role involves in-depth skills and knowledge to effectively manage the care of a client population. The nurse in the case manager role may assume responsibility for providing nursing care to the client, or may carry out additional aspects of case management while arranging for other nurses to provide the necessary care.

As a *technology*, case management generates tools and techniques to organize care. These technologies maximize the timing and sequencing of multiple, often complex, care activities.

As a *process*, case management expands on the components of the nursing process: assessment, goal/outcome development, planning, intervention, monitoring, and evaluation. The unique feature of case management is that it is episode-focused, viewing health issues and responding to the care needs of clients along the illness and/or care continuum (often across multiple settings), rather than being confined to the provision of care within one setting.

There are multiple primary goals for case management: optimizing the client's self-care capabilities, promoting the efficient use of resources, and stimulating the creation of new services. Additional goals include providing quality care along a continuum, decreasing the fragmentation of care across many settings, enhancing the client's quality of life, and cost containment. These goals are often achieved through preventing inappropriate institutionalization or delaying institutionalization in acute and long-term settings. Case management promotes the provision of quality care in the least restrictive environment. Other terms for case management include "service management," "care coordination," and "care management." As explained earlier in this section, "managed care" is not another term for case management, but is a different concept focusing on system-wide utilization controls, rather than on individual clients.

As a *service*, case management provides both facilitating and gatekeeping functions for the client. Many clients and their informal caregivers can neither access nor unravel the health care delivery system to their best advantage. As noted by the National Council on Aging (1987), case management helps clients and caregivers make informed decisions based on the client's needs, abilities, resources, and personal preferences. Case management also can personalize care in an otherwise impersonal system. The case manager considers the client's health status and diagnoses, treatment plans, payment resources, and health care options. There are increasing opportunities for clients and caregivers to seek out and purchase case management services. This is particularly true for families with elder-care responsibilities.

The access/facilitation service of case management assures that clients receive appropriate, individualized, and cost-effective care within a system of services. Many clients who are members of managed care systems, such as HMOs and PPOs, and clients with various private insurance arrangements are automatically enrolled in a case management program when they experience certain types of health crises (such as head injuries), as part of cost-containment efforts.

Case management, however, is still evolving. Nurses in the case manager role address the issues of allocation of resources, effectiveness of care, and cost containment. Nurses who practice as case managers or who integrate case management into their practice are introducing new professional dimensions within institutions and in private practice.

Further, as a vital component of the health care system, case management can encompass the conceptual framework of individual practitioners and facilitate personal practice model developments in nursing. In addition to the valuable service it provides the client, case management has the potential to increase the nurse's level of satisfaction and sense of autonomy as a health care provider.

Historical Perspective

Community service coordination, a forerunner of case management, began at the turn of the century in public health programs, and providing service coordination has always been a focus of public health nursing (Grau, 1984). The Visiting Nurse Service was one of the very first community health programs (Stanhope and Lancaster, 1984). Service coordination has since evolved into case management, but case management considerably expands upon coordination of community services.

The concept of a continuum of care was used after World War II to describe the extended community services necessary to provide care for discharged psychiatric patients (Grau, 1984). The term "case management" first appeared in the early 1970s in social welfare literature (Stanhope and Lancaster, 1984), followed by many articles in nursing literature.

In recent years, the U.S. government has moved to establish health care programs that focus on a comprehensive, coordinated continuum of care at the community level, by implementing several research and demonstration projects. One of the first of these was the Triage Project, which began in Connecticut in 1974 as an effort to test the feasibility, cost, and effectiveness of a client-centered model for health care delivery.

Other early programs that were established on the city, county, or state levels include the Georgia Alternative Health Services, Monroe County Community Long-Term Care, Wisconsin Coordinated Care for the Disabled, New York Long-Term Home Health Care, and San Francisco's On Lok Community Care for Dependent Adults (Stanhope and Lancaster, 1984).

The 1981 Omnibus Budget Reconciliation Act and Medicare prospective reimbursement encouraged community-based alternatives to institutional placement. Federal demonstration projects also linked case management to long-term community care of the aged. These programs were designed to provide and evaluate comprehensive, coordinated services.

Other programs were funded by grants from state governments and private foundations. In some cases, Medicare and Medicaid waivers were sought in order to provide funding for services not yet approved by Medicare and Medicaid. These waivers allowed greater numbers of consumers access to needed services. In essence, the system was adapted to meet the needs of the client.

In the private sector, insurers have become increasingly concerned about the rising costs of health care. In the 1980s, commercial insurance companies, HMOs, PPOs, and workers' compensation programs, as well as the industries purchasing their services, identified the need to more carefully coordinate and manage the care of clients within "catastrophic" case types. Thus, case management has sometimes been implemented as a strategy to simultaneously coordinate care and manage the costs of particularly expensive, resource-intensive cases.

Historically, nurses have recognized the need for case management and welcomed the opportunities to learn the necessary skills. Health care activities may change with technology, but the goals remain the same: to reduce the incidence of disease, premature death, discomfort, and disability, and to increase or maintain health and the quality of life. Nurses' leadership in case management reflects nursing's tradition of coordinating various resources to meet clients' multiple service needs.

Why Case Management?

Case management addresses a wide variety of health care issues and needs. As a result, it is often implemented for multiple reasons, including:

1. Case management focuses on the full spectrum of needs presented by clients and their families; it is client-focused. Client and family satisfaction within case- managed systems is generally high.
2. A strong component of case management is an outcome orientation to care. The goal is to move with the client/family toward optimal care outcomes.
3. Case management facilitates and promotes coordination of client care, minimizing fragmentation.
4. Case management promotes cost-effective care by minimizing fragmentation, maximizing coordination, and facilitating client/family movement through the health care system.
5. Case management maximizes and coordinates the contributions of all disciplines within the health care team.

6. Case management responds to the needs of insurers and other third-party payers, specifically those related to outcome-based, cost-effective care.
7. The needs of clients, providers, and payers all receive attention within a case management system. Case management represents a merger of clinical and financial interests, systems, and outcomes.
8. Case management can be included in the marketing strategies of hospitals and other institutions to target clients/families, insurers, and employers.

These eight characteristics of case management further serve to differentiate it from managed care. The client/family focus; the coordination of services provided by various health care disciplines; the merging of patient, clinical, and financial concerns; and the ability to market case management services to interested parties are not characteristics shared by managed care arrangements. Case management's focus on individual clients and their care is unique.

In choosing to move toward a case management model, it is imperative that the initial, desired goals for such a change be defined. These goals or outcomes will affect the ultimate design of the case management model, as well as serve as a baseline against which future progress can be assessed.

Who Should Receive Case Management Services?

Case management is an effective strategy for selected client populations. In most programs, case management is applied to priority client groups rather than all clients, given the expense sometimes associated with a coordinated case management program.

Clients are usually selected for case management programs within the parameters of high cost, high volume, and/or high risk criteria. For example, case management programs may be directed toward "catastrophic" case types (such as patients with head injuries, AIDS patients, transplants, or neonates). Case management can facilitate access to needed services and coordinate care for clients within the fragmented health care delivery system, prevent avoidable episodes of illness among at-risk clients, and control or reduce the cost of care borne by the client or third-party payers.

Many case managers work with broad client populations. Alternatively, however, some case managers may focus on specific populations, such as clients grouped by presenting or principal diagnosis, diagnosis-related group (DRG), age, nursing diagnosis, physician, payer, or within the acute-chronic continuum.

Three identifiable groups of clients provide examples of case-managed populations. The first group consists of frail, chronically disabled clients who are functionally or emotionally impaired. Many of these clients are over 85 years of age. Others who may be in this category include, but are not limited to, the developmentally disabled, physically handicapped, and mentally handicapped.

The second group of clients consists of those with long-term, medically complex problems requiring multifaceted, costly care. This group includes, but is not limited to, high-risk infants, individuals who have HIV infection or AIDS, clients with transplants, and individuals who are dependent upon technology.

The third group is made up of clients who are severely compromised by an acute episode of illness or an acute exacerbation of a chronic illness.

Rights of Clients

Certain rights should be observed for all case management clients. A task force of the National Council on Aging (1987) recommended the following as basic client rights in case management services:

- The right to be given a fair and comprehensive assessment of his or her health and functional, psychosocial, and cognitive abilities.
- The right to have access to needed health and social services.
- The right to be treated with respect and dignity.
- The right to self-determination, including the opportunity to participate in developing a plan for services.
- The right to privacy and confidentiality.
- The right to know the cost of services prior to their being rendered, especially in cases where the client will be responsible for payment.

- The right to be notified of any change of service, termination of service, or discharge from the program.
- The right to withdraw from the case management program at any time that he or she is dissatisfied with the case management service being given.
- The right to a grievance procedure in the event that the client feels his or her rights have been violated, or perceives discrimination or inappropriate treatment.

Designing Case Management Programs

The Nurse as Client Advocate

Case management provides an opportunity for nurses to act as advocates for their clients. Nurses focus on providing the most cost-effective referrals to a broad range of appropriate providers, as well as promoting, restoring, and maintaining client health. Case management by nurses has the potential to increase consumer responsibility, as well as to increase the consumer's role in health care decision making. The intended focus on partnerships between consumers enables nurses to ensure that health services are appropriate, effective, cost-effective, and focused on consumer needs (Nursing's Agenda for Health Care Reform, 1991).

Appreciating the Diversity

Because case management is a process, there are multiple approaches to and models for its operationalization. Case management is operationalized within a variety of contexts, patient populations, and settings — a factor contributing to its diversity. In short, there is no "one way" to do case management. The context, purpose, objectives, and scope are integral to designing case management programs. In turn, these factors are influential when designing role functions. Schwartz, Goldman, and Churgin (1982) describe the term "case management" as a Rorschach test, suggesting that an organization would project onto case management its own particular goals and priorities.

There are multiple variables and questions to consider in designing case management programs and roles, including:

- What is the scope and nature of the client population to be case managed? Are the clients chronically or acutely ill? Are their health problems single-episode by nature, or will cyclic interventions be required? What is the client population's socioeconomic profile? Who are the principal payers associated with the case-managed clients?
- Where is the case manager's role based — in the acute care setting, in the community, as a component of third-party payers, or within a social agency?
- Are the case managers also the providers of direct client care, or is their focus on the coordination of care provided by others?
- What are the primary goals of the case management program?
- Is the nature of the case management program envisioned as primarily clinical, administrative, or a blend of both?

The answers to these questions shape the design of the case management program and should be carefully considered before finalizing the model.

Characteristics of Case Management Programs

Case management programs exhibit a number of characteristics that serve as distinguishing features:

- Case management is episode-based — it does not exclusively focus on the care provided within one area. Case managers are attentive to the care needs of clients across a continuum of settings and phases. This promotes continuity of the plan and provider across the continuum for as much of the episode of illness as possible.
- Case management is longitudinally-based. It follows a client across the continuum of illness and refers the client to the most appropriate provider. This promotes effective utilization of the health care system and provides for an optimum level of rehabilitation/ restoration.
- Typically, case management programs are directed toward targeted or selected client populations. Clients are usually admitted into case management programs from high-cost, high-volume, or high-risk categories.

- Case management focuses on coordinating services and transitions. It puts the pieces together.
- Case management programs are quality (outcome) driven.
- Case management programs are fiscally aware and responsive, and work to strengthen the cost-quality link for clients and organizations. Management of the costs of care is an important role function for case managers.
- Clients and their families are the central focus of case management programs, as case managers:
  - Consider the full range of needs and issues presented.
  - Advocate for clients and their families.
  - Foster decision making, independence, and growth.
  - Establish an effective relationship with the client/family nucleus.
  - Educate clients/families and support them in moving toward self-care.
- Collaboration is an essential characteristic, since case management taps into the expertise of many disciplines. To be successful, case managers must secure the input, cooperation, and active involvement of all providers essential to the care of the identified client population.
- In many case management programs, the ability to procure and enhance the accessibility of services is a benchmark.
- Case management programs are proactive — preventing problems and issues, and interrupting cyclic patterns.

Who Should Be a Case Manager?

The question of who best functions in the case manager role is controversial, focusing on:

- Whether the individual in the case manager role should be a clinician or a professional, or whether paraprofessional staff are capable of fulfilling the role.
- Whether nurses are the ideal candidates for the case manager role, or whether other disciplines are equally effective in this role.

To respond to these issues, it is important to reexamine the context, nature, and scope of the case management program. Schwartz, Goldman, and Churgin (1982) provide a persuasive argument that case managers should have a clinical background, observing that:

> Although they may not provide direct clinical service, good case managers require substantial clinical knowledge, skills, and judgment. When fiscal control is only minimally linked to clinical sophistication, case managers may be able to ensure that their clients' needs are met, but they may not be capable of determining what those needs really are.

Responding to the issue of whether nurses are the ideal case managers, Grau (1984) observes:

> Most policy makers and practitioners agree that case management is not a profession, but a set of functions to be carried out by persons capable of doing so.... For the client, the nature of the case manager's background is important. It influences the kind of direct care the case manager provides as well as other aspects of service delivery and monitoring. The critical factor in determining who fills the case manager role is the nature of the population to be served.

Nurses are particularly suited to provide case management for clients with multiple health problems that have a health-related component. *Nursing: A Social Policy Statement* (American Nurses Association, 1980) describes the nature of nursing as complex and highly interactive — two elements that also describe case management. The social policy statement depicts nursing as a nurturing discipline, focused more on creating the physiological, psychological, and sociocultural environment in which the client can gain or maintain health than on the diagnosis and treatment of disease. These characteristics of nursing demonstrate why nurses are adept at providing case management; that is, assisting the client to negotiate in today's health care system.

Nurses bring broad-based and unique skills and knowledge to case management. The role of the nurse as a coordinator of care has been integral to defining nursing practice for decades. The coordination of services and care is the primary function of case managers. This role is a logical extension of the nursing role. Case management is usually described as attending to the total needs and concerns presented by clients and their families. Nurses focus on assisting and facilitating clients as they adapt to the potential or actual effects of health issues on daily activities — another integral component of the case manager role. Within a holistic perspective, nurses practice with extensive knowledge of the multifaceted issues presented by clients and their families, while including the physical and psychosocial dimensions. This is particularly true of nurses' abilities to assess both the initial and changing health status and needs of their clients. The skills and knowledge that nurses bring to the case management role are unique when compared to other disciplines, such as social service or physical therapy. Nurses have skills and knowledge that extend beyond the biophysical and pathological aspects of care, bringing a holistic perspective and knowledge base to the care of case-managed clients.

Mundinger (1984) summarizes the arguments that support nurses in case manager roles by noting that, "Nurses can provide the majority of services that social workers offer to these clients, but the converse is not true; social workers have few, if any, of the physical assessment or illness detections skills of the nurse." Appointing nurses to the case manager role ensures a more complete "fit" between the skills of the nurse and the needs of the role and case-managed clients.

Another controversial issue is generated by physicians who propose that they are the only case managers for their clients. In a case management program, physicians are the managers of the medical plan of care. However, it is increasingly evident that medical care is but one dimension within the total picture of patient care. The other dimensions must be carefully coordinated for maximum effectiveness and efficiency, and must be integrated with the physician's plan of care to minimize fragmentation and disruption of service. Case managers can facilitate the physician's plan of care and minimize interruptions to the ideal timing and sequencing within the care system.

For many client populations, an ideal case management model may be a multidisciplinary group practice that incorporates members from each of the disciplines involved in the care of a specified client population. The members are formally appointed to the group practice and coordinate (and in some instances provide) care for client populations along the continuum of health care settings. The nursing members of the group practice modality are the core of the practice and represent each setting where nursing care is provided to the case-managed population. Group practice case management is effective because the members establish effective communication systems among themselves; focus on the "ideal practice" for the client population; provide early identification and continuity of care for client and family issues; and effect changes within the system and among providers that enhance quality, satisfaction, and cost-effectiveness. The client subsequently perceives that there is a well-organized group providing a broad spectrum of services and care.

Nursing Case Management

As noted earlier, case management is a generic term that is becoming increasingly diversified. Nursing case management is emerging as a branch or model of generic case management. This model tends to be clinically-oriented, although administrative aspects (particularly cost containment) are also a major role function. Nursing departments within health care organizations (e.g., hospitals, rehabilitation facilities, Visiting Nurse Associations) have turned to nursing case management as a means to improve the quality of care delivery, empower nurses, and facilitate the attainment of institutional and departmental goals for cost-effectiveness. These agency- or institution-based models are often described as internal case management programs, differing from external case management programs or programs which are administered by agencies other than the provider institution (e.g., insurance companies or HMO case management programs). Use of these external programs of case management is often triggered by the onset of a particularly catastrophic health event, such as severe head trauma, which may entail expensive, long-term rehabilitative care and case management.

Nursing case management is based on the premise that client care must be carefully coordinated across the continuum of care settings, including the client's needs for nursing care. Although the nurses in the case manager role may be based in one setting, they usually have influence or input into the care of their case-managed clients in other settings. Nursing care is one of the elements of client care that has become increasingly fragmented within recent years. This is related to factors such as the decreasing use of primary nursing and the tendency of nurses to specialize within one particular care setting — such as the emergency department, intensive care unit, or ambulatory clinic — which can impair their understanding and vision of the care provided to clients in other settings across the continuum. The specialized nature of the nursing work force is one of the factors which further indicate that an identified manager of nursing care is needed. Nursing case management is one such approach to alleviating the issues and effects of fragmentation.

Nurse case managers have a broad vision of client care needs, especially as they relate to desired outcomes. They support patients in moving toward those outcomes within the continuum of care represented by the client populations. Nurse case managers are sensitive to the issues of costs of care for both the client and the institution within which they function. In this context, the role of the case manager is constantly evolving and differentiating from the role of general nurse clinicians.

Nurse case managers often incorporate direct care as a part of their role, although the percentage of time they spend in direct care varies between programs. As they provide and coordinate the care of case-managed clients, nurse case managers are attentive to opportunities for creating changes in system and clinician practices that will both improve and streamline care. They may function as members of a group practice or as individual managers of care.

This emerging model of case management demonstrates that the improved coordination of the nursing care provided to clients (especially within discharge planning and teaching), when integrated and coordinated with the care provided by other disciplines, is a very powerful strategy for producing effective, efficient quality care.

Other potential issues need to be recognized and addressed when designing nursing case management systems. Ideally, nursing case management streamlines the process of coordinating patient care. However, another layer can be added to the process. Nursing case management can be an effective vehicle for empowering nurses. Power is not present within roles or organizations in limited quantities. However, the effect of a particular role design may be the empowerment of a nursing group (such as the case managers) at the cost of disenfranchising another group (such as staff nurses).

To minimize the risk of these potential issues, roles and their interfaces among staff nurses and case managers need to be defined as clearly as possible when the case management model is designed. Ideally, a nursing case management model empowers all members of the nursing team, along with other members of the multidisciplinary team, and ultimately, the clients and families served. Nursing case management needs to be integrated into the organizational structure, rather than merely added to the existing design.

Additionally, nursing case management is not a solution for all of the identified problems and issues within the nursing profession or within the health care system. In fact, the implementation of nursing case management can emphasize previously existing issues or problems, particularly those associated with the underlying nursing care delivery system. Nursing case management is not a nursing care delivery system. Throughout the history of nursing, four nursing care delivery systems have emerged — functional, team, total patient care, and primary. These models can be modified and integrated to meet the needs of the setting; however, nursing case management is not such a system.

Nursing care delivery systems generally apply to all patients within a given area or institution, are unit-based in terms of patient care focus, and provide a framework regarding the patient care assignments of various nursing personnel. Conversely, nursing case management generally focuses on specifically identified patient populations (high-risk, high- volume, high-cost), addresses care needs across the episode or continuum of an illness, and often identifies how personnel assignments will be made. Nursing case management may, in fact, indicate a need to reexamine and revise how nursing care is provided to all patients within the organization. It can increase the accountability of staff nurses, as well as the case managers.

Core Components and Role Functions in Case Management

The specific activities of the case manager blend with the stages of the nursing process or clinical reasoning process to form a framework for nursing case management (Nursing Assessment and Management of the Frail Elderly Project, 1987).

Interact

The interaction essential to case management requires the development of relationships among the nurse case manager, client, family members, and other service providers. Trust and support are built through effective communication techniques that foster relationships among the client, family, nurse case manager, and other providers of care central to the entire case management process.

The interaction component of nursing case management involves the tasks of case-finding and screening. The main purposes of the initial screening include outlining the problem, determining the need for case management services, and determining the client's eligibility for services. If the client is not eligible for case management according to preestablished guidelines, he or she is referred for assistance as appropriate. It is imperative that the case manager be knowledgeable about the community resources available.

Assess: Establish a Data Base

The assessment component of case management allows a comprehensive evaluation to be made of the client's physical health status, functional capability, mental status, personal and community support systems, financial resources, and environmental conditions. Standardized assessment instruments are often used to obtain this comprehensive data base. Standardized instruments facilitate the collection of both individual and aggregate data. The comprehensive functional assessment of clients is frequently performed by an interdisciplinary team consisting of a nurse, a social worker, and, at times, other professionals.

The multiplicity of problems and the complexity of services for high-risk clients, such as the frail elderly, premature infants, and the developmentally disabled, make providing them with case management a challenge. An assessment interview in the client's home environment to determine strengths and areas for concern can be vital to the overall planning process. However, the point of contact may be within the hospital or other health care setting. During the assessment process, the nurse and other team members work with the client and/or significant others to mutually determine the problems, strengths, and needs of the client. After the data are collected, they are analyzed and synthesized to arrive at nursing diagnoses and/or interdisciplinary problem statements.

Plan

The next phase of the case management process is developing the service care plan with client participation. Essential components of this phase include setting mutually agreed-upon goals with measurable objectives; determining action steps toward goal achievement; and enumerating and selecting essential resources and services through collaboration among health care professionals, the client, and the family or significant others. By the conclusion of this phase, the nurse case manager, other professionals, the client, and the family have developed a care plan that designates the needs that can be addressed through informal support systems and those for which formal services will be required.

Implement

The fourth phase of the case management process, implementation, aims to provide for the delivery of care by linking the client with appropriate service providers. In some models of case management, the nurse is both a provider of direct nursing care and the coordinator of services. In other models, the nurse in the case manager role serves only as a coordinator, and direct care is provided by other professional nurses.

Formal contracts and agreements are sometimes established between the case manager or case management firm and health care providers. Throughout the implementation phase, the case manager coordinates care so that the client and health care providers clearly understand and fulfill their part in the service care plan.

During the implementation phase, the case manager is frequently called upon to advocate on behalf of the client. Client advocacy often involves providing additional information and education about conflict resolution and how to prevent denial of services or denial of financing of services for which the client is eligible, and extension of services already in place. The case manager also identifies gaps in the service continuum and advocates for needed changes in the community.

Finally, the case manager must provide for education of the client, family, and significant others concerning the importance of self-care by the client. Self-care at the highest level of functioning is essential to the client's sense of autonomy and self-determination.

Evaluate

The final phase of the case management process is monitoring and evaluation. During this phase, the case manager maintains contact with the client, the client's informal support systems, and direct service providers in order to continually evaluate the client's responses to interventions and his or her progress toward preestablished goals.

The client data base may change over time, requiring some revisions of the problem statements or nursing diagnoses, and modifications of the goals based on the ongoing assessment of the client and the environment. Ongoing care coordination is necessary until outcomes are achieved. The client may be discharged or assigned to inactive status as appropriate. The outcomes, both expected and unexpected, must be evaluated. In addition, there must be a quality improvement program for ongoing systematic monitoring and evaluation of the case management program. The services delivered by providers and subcontractors as a result of case management activities also must be evaluated through a quality improvement program. When cost containment is being vigorously pursued, as in the current health care environment, it is particularly important to monitor the quality of care in the client's interest. Professional standards, such as those published by the American Nurses Association (1974, 1982,

1983, 1986a, 1986b, 1987c, 1987d, 1991), provide a basis for developing quality management activities.

Role Functions

As noted earlier, a case manager's tasks and the ensuing priorities differ according to the organizational setting, the target population, and the nature of the practice (whether it involves only coordination of services, or both coordination activities and direct delivery of nursing care). Despite variations in the case manager role, certain skills and functions appropriate to most case manager positions can be identified. Primary functions include, but are not limited to, the following:

- Coordinating care and services, including coordination of care and service providers responsible for furnishing services needed by a given client and, in many models, of all payment sources that reimburse providers for those services.
- Case-finding and screening to identify appropriate clients for case management.
- Comprehensively assessing the client's goals, as well as his or her physical, functional, psychological, social, environmental, and financial statuses.
- Assessing the client's informal and formal support systems.
- Analyzing and synthesizing all data for formulating appropriate nursing diagnoses and/or interdisciplinary problem statements.
- Developing, implementing, monitoring, and modifying a plan of care through an interdisciplinary and collaborative team process, in conjunction with the client and his or her caregivers.
- Linking the client with the most appropriate institutional or community resource, advocating on behalf of the client for scarce resources, and developing new resources if gaps exist in the service continuum.
- Procuring services, including eligibility decisions and authorizing hospitalization and home care (essential in some programs).
- Problem solving.
- Facilitating access.
- Providing direct patient care, in some programs.
- Providing liaison services.

- Educating the client, the family, and community support services; facilitating the goal of self-care by the client and his or her family.
- Facilitating communication.
- Documenting.
- Monitoring the client's progress toward goal achievement and periodically reassessing changes in health status.
- Monitoring the plan to ensure the quality, quantity, timeliness, and effectiveness of services; providing periodic reassessment to assure that services are appropriate, cost-effective, and not increasing the client's dependence.
- Monitoring activities to ensure that services are actually being delivered and meet the needs of the client.
- Evaluating client and program outcomes to determine whether the client should be discharged or assigned inactive status.

The primary focus of the case manager role varies among programs. However, there is a general consensus that the principal role or function of case managers is that of coordinator of care and services. This function is the basis for all other aspects of the case management role.

Other questions arise when designing case manager roles. For example, dilemmas about defining authority, accountability, and interrelationships might arise. The authority issue demands defining the parameters within which case managers operate and outlining the scope of their influence. Case managers often wield four kinds of authority—administrative, legal, fiscal, and clinical (Schwartz, Goldman, and Churgin, 1982). The accountability factor defines the scope of influence and practice: within the program, what is the case manager accountable for and to whom? The latter question, to whom is the case manager accountable, raises the issue of defining interrelationships within the program, including the identification of formal and informal associations.

Defining a Knowledge Base for Case Management

Nurses assuming the case manager role require in-depth knowledge and skills. These requirements are generic, transcending the issues of where or by whom the case manager is employed. The knowledge and skills essential to functioning as a case manager are outlined in this section. These skills and knowledge sets can be used to develop a curriculum for new case managers, as well as to establish parameters for prioritizing qualified candidates for the case manager role.

- In-depth knowledge of the health care financial environment. This encompasses a working knowledge of the principles and effects of DRGs, HMOs, PPOs, and other financial systems. Case managers also must be knowledgeable about the financial dimensions of the client populations they manage. An in-depth, working knowledge of the particular requirements and parameters established by clients' third-party payers is essential, particularly within case management programs administered by insurance companies.
- In-depth clinical knowledge and skills. Because case management is attentive to clients' needs across the continuum of care, knowledge of the current advances in each care arena (such as home, inpatient, or rehabilitation care) is vital. In addition, case managers need enhanced skills in the nursing process, with particular expertise in the assessment and outcome (or goal development) dimensions. Assessment-related skills are, to some degree, dependent on the nature and context of the case manager's role. However, it is imperative that case managers have the skill to establish baseline information about the client's health status, psychosocial issues, and sources of support. Case management functions also emphasize the need for skills in developing realistic goals or outcomes, especially in light of the complex physical and psychosocial needs presented by case-managed clients. These clinical skills enable case managers to establish more effective sequencing and timing of care activities, ultimately reducing fragmentation and costs. They also contribute to the case manager's ability to think critically and make sound clinical judgments.
- Care resources for case-managed clients within both the institution and the community. This dimension includes knowledge about current community resources and how to access them effectively and efficiently. Within advanced case management skills exists the possibility of facilitating and supporting the development of new resources and supports to meet changing client needs.

- Discharge planning, including the ideal timing and sequencing of discharge-related activities, as well as in-depth knowledge of the care requirements of clients in various settings (such as home or extended care).
- Management skills, including communication, delegation, negotiation and persuasion, sources and uses of power, consultation, problem-solving, meeting management, conflict management, confrontation, negotiating and managing change, technical writing, networking, marketing, priority setting, time management, group development, human resource development, accountability, authority, advocacy, ethical decision- making, and project management.
- Collaboration and effective team strategies.
- Teaching, counseling, and education skills — focusing on patients/families, peers, and other members of the health care team. The pacing, sequencing, and appropriateness of patient education content is of particular concern.
- Program evaluation and research.
- Quality improvement strategies and techniques.
- The process of role development and negotiation.
- Peer consultation and evaluation.
- The requirements and eligibility parameters for services established by the client's third-party payer and by governmental agencies.

A formal orientation program assists new case managers to develop or enhance their skills and knowledge in the areas outlined above. The ongoing development of case management skills is facilitated through forums such as regular case discussion and review, peer consultation, participation in local and national programs, performance appraisal (including the process of self-evaluation), and group problem-solving sessions. Because the case manager role is constantly evolving, it is imperative that some or all of these forums be made available on a regular and formal basis.

In addition to the skills and knowledge domains outlined above, ideal case manager candidates demonstrate several characteristics which also can be used in identifying candidates who are likely to excel in the case manager role. These characteristics include team participation, risk taking, clinical maturity, critical thinking, creativity, tenacity, goal orientation, enthusiasm, commitment, optimal self-care, and a sense of humor.

Educational Preparation

The American Nurses Association recommends that the minimum preparation for a nurse case manager is a baccalaureate in nursing with three years of appropriate clinical experience. This preparation is in accord with requirements outlined in *The Scope of Nursing Practice* (American Nurses Association, 1987b), which identifies the baccalaureate as preparation for the full scope of the clinical practice of nursing. It also is consistent with guidelines presented in *Standards of Community Health Nursing Practice* (American Nurses Association, 1986a), *Standards of Home Health Nursing Practice* (American Nurses Association, 1986b), and *Standards and Scope of Gerontological Nursing Practice* (American Nurses Association, 1987c), which describe coordination of services and case management as a function of the nurse generalist.

Although the baccalaureate in nursing is the minimum educational preparation required for case managers, many existing case management programs prefer master's-prepared nurses who are experienced clinical nurse specialists in areas related to the target population, and who have worked in the types of service settings the case manager is most likely to encounter.

In an attempt to meet this educational need, a model curriculum for nurse case managers in community-based long-term care of the elderly was developed and is currently being tested over a five-year period by faculty at the University of Kansas School of Nursing, Kansas City, Kansas.

The concepts of Orem's (1980) self-care model were integrated throughout the Nursing Assessment and Management of the Frail Elderly (NAMFE) curriculum to maximize the self-care potential of the individual, the family, and the community. The University of Kansas course consists of eight learning modules that provide a systematic approach to the comprehensive functional assessment and care coordination of the frail elderly residing in the community. [The specific content of the eight NAMFE modules is presented in the Appendix at the end of this book.]

The NAMFE course in Kansas is a statewide continuing education program for gerontological and community health nurses. It is anticipated that the NAMFE model curriculum, with appropriate leveling of the content, may assist schools of nursing to integrate additional case management knowledge and skills into existing undergraduate and graduate curricula.

Thus far, the concepts of case management have been integrated into the curriculum design of various other programs, including the Vanderbilt University School of Nursing, which grants the master of science in nursing as the first professional degree.

Effects of Case Management Programs

Case management has demonstrated effectiveness in lowering costs and improving client outcomes and satisfaction. The case management role allows nurses to more concretely and visibly contribute to institutional and/or programmatic goals related to cost-effectiveness. The cost savings are related to various factors, including:

- Enhanced communication with and education of clients and their families, enabling them to better plan for and make more fully informed decisions about care.
- Earlier identification of discharge needs (often before an inpatient admission), resulting in the development of plans to address potential or real barriers.
- Identification of patient problems and barriers to care within a time frame that allows them to be addressed proactively or concurrently, rather than retrospectively.
- More effective and efficient communication among the disciplines involved in client care, as well as with clients and their families.
- Reduction or elimination of duplicate or overlapping care, tests, and treatments through improved sequencing and coordination of care activities.
- Minimized or eliminated delays in required tests, treatments, or care.
- Enhanced knowledge among clinicians regarding the financial aspects of care.
- Attention to the needs of clients and the issues and problems encountered in providing efficient, effective care at both the individual and aggregate client levels. Addressing the issues encountered in the care of aggregate groups of clients provides the case manager with useful data that can facilitate system changes that improve the cost and quality of care.

The financial outcomes of case management reflect the tenet that quality care is cost-effective care. Several evaluation studies, including the models presented herein, attest to this fact.

A bedside case management approach at Logan Regional Hospital in Utah has achieved a 40 percent reduction in the difference between costs incurred by the patient and costs reimbursed by capitated payment systems on 10 targeted diagnosis-related groups (Bair, Griswold and Head, 1989).

The New England Medical Center, a 470-bed Boston teaching hospital, has reduced lengths of stay by one day for many patients, and cut costs by as much as 40 percent in major clinical departments through the use of a detailed case management system.

A frequently cited study concerns the professional nurse case manager role at the hub of the nursing HMO at Carondelet St. Mary's Hospital in Tucson, Arizona (Ethridge, 1991). Cost data have indicated that some chronically-ill patients were not hospitalized at all because of the effective intervention of the professional nurse case manager. The immediate access to health care, which nurse case managers provide, decreased patients' lengths of stay and, therefore, decreased costs of hospitalization.

Another study assessing the cost-effectiveness of case management, using a quasi-experimental design on 128 cesarean section patients, demonstrated a decrease in length of stay and an improvement in patient recovery time (Cohen, 1991). Incorporated in this case management model were clinical practice outcome measures described as critical pathways. The potential savings for one year were determined to be $1,095,080.80.

Pittman (1989) described the positive impact of case management on the deinstitutionalization of the chronically mentally ill. Case management has helped clients make informed decisions about their health care and has provided a personalized approach within the bureaucracy of health care.

Positive patient experiences also were demonstrated by Joachim (1989), using the school nurse as case manager for chronically-ill children. By utilizing a collaborative approach with teachers, school officials, classmates, and parents, resources for these children were maximized to create a positive school environment and academic experience.

In addition to cost-effectiveness, another benefit of case management is that nurses express satisfaction in the case manager role; a number of factors contribute. Case management provides an opportunity for nurses to utilize the full scope of their education and experience, and challenges them to expand their knowledge and skills. Case management also empowers nurses, placing them in pivotal positions to manage the quality and cost of health care. Reward and recognition systems may be enhanced in a case management system. Nurses in this role find that collegiality and collaboration with other disciplines is strengthened.

An additional benefit of case management is that clients and their families find case managed care satisfying. In many programs, the case manager role is designed to promote an effective relationship with individual clients. Clients sense that care is organized and coordinated by various disciplines. This promotes a sense of security and satisfaction. Within the advocacy component of case management, clients know that they have an identified individual (or group) to whom they can turn as issues arise.

Prior to the implementation of DRGs, the Long-Term Care Demonstration Project of 1982-83 (Caragno et al., 1986) clearly showed the effect of quality nursing care. With the evolution of the science of nursing, as well as improvements in case management by nurses, quality care remains a focus within a demonstrated cost-containment atmosphere. The following models of case management attest to this fact. The models selected for inclusion herein are intended to be descriptive; they constitute neither an all-inclusive set of models nor a representative sample of case management programs. It is hoped that these models will stimulate further use of case management by nurses with clients whose care is multifaceted.

Case Management Models

Carondelet St. Mary's Hospital and Health Center Model*

Carondelet St. Mary's Hospital and Health Center has 374 acute care beds and provides a full continuum of health and nursing services, including hospice, home health, and 14 nurse- managed community health centers. Carondelet St. Mary's is located in Tucson, Arizona, an urban community with diverse social and ethnic groups, including large Hispanic and Native American populations. A professional practice model of nursing with shared governance, acuity-based billing for nursing care, and salaried status has been in place for many years. The foundation for the professional practice model reflects a holistic framework that emphasizes respect for clients' choices and the importance of working in partnership with others (Ethridge, 1991).

In 1986, Carondelet St. Mary's created a nursing case management program in response to the profound changes occurring nationally in the health care system. In this program, hospital-based nurse case managers work with high-risk individuals across the health care continuum, spending about 30 percent of their time inside, and 70 percent of their time outside the hospital. The nurse case managers work in partnership with their clients to assist them in managing their health care needs and in accessing necessary community health care support services.

The nurse case managers typically begin their work with clients during hospitalization. With the assistance of the acute care nursing

*From Gerri S. Lamb, Ph.D., R.N., Clinical Director for Research, Professional Nurse Case Manager, Carondelet St. Mary's Hospital and Health Center, Tucson, Arizona. Reprinted with permission.

staff and other members of the health care team, they identify individuals who may be unable to manage their care at home or who are at risk for recurrent hospitalizations. These often are older adults who are cognitively or emotionally challenged, who have inadequate supports in the community, or who are predisposed to sudden physiological imbalance. The clients often have chronic cardiovascular or respiratory diseases and have patterns of frequent emergency department or hospital use during acute exacerbations of their disease. The nurse case mangers establish a long-term relationship with these individuals, and work with them across health care settings between and during exacerbations. As the individuals' needs match their eligibility for programs and services, the nurse case manager directs them to appropriate nursing and health care services available at Carondelet St. Mary's and in the Tucson community.

A second group of clients nurse case managers commonly work with includes older adults experiencing acute illnesses, such as myocardial infarctions or fractured hips. Often, these clients may not be homebound or need skilled nursing after discharge and, therefore, are not eligible for Medicare-reimbursed home health services. However, they may need transitional assistance in managing their illness or injury and in regaining personal or family balance if they are to remain in the community and avoid repeated hospitalizations or long-term skilled care placement.

The nurse case managers at Carondelet St. Mary's are part of a system of nursing services called the Professional Nursing Network (see Figure 1). Within the network, individuals have access to a full range of nursing services, including acute, rehabilitation, home health, long-term, community/primary, and hospice nursing care. The nurse case manager links the client to a primary nurse in these systems and facilitates smooth transitions and continuity of care. Since individuals may need short-term or long-term assistance, the frequency and duration of nursing case management services are tailored to the individual situation, and are negotiated between the nurse case manager and the client. The nurse case managers may work for weeks or months with clients undergoing sudden, acute illnesses, who often are only at high risk temporarily for adverse outcomes. In contrast, the nurse case managers may work for several months or even years with chronically ill individuals who experience frequent exacerbations or who are gradually entering the terminal phases of their disease.

The minimum degree held by nurse case managers at Carondelet St. Mary's is the baccalaureate in nursing. Several individuals who

Figure 1
The Professional Nursing Network

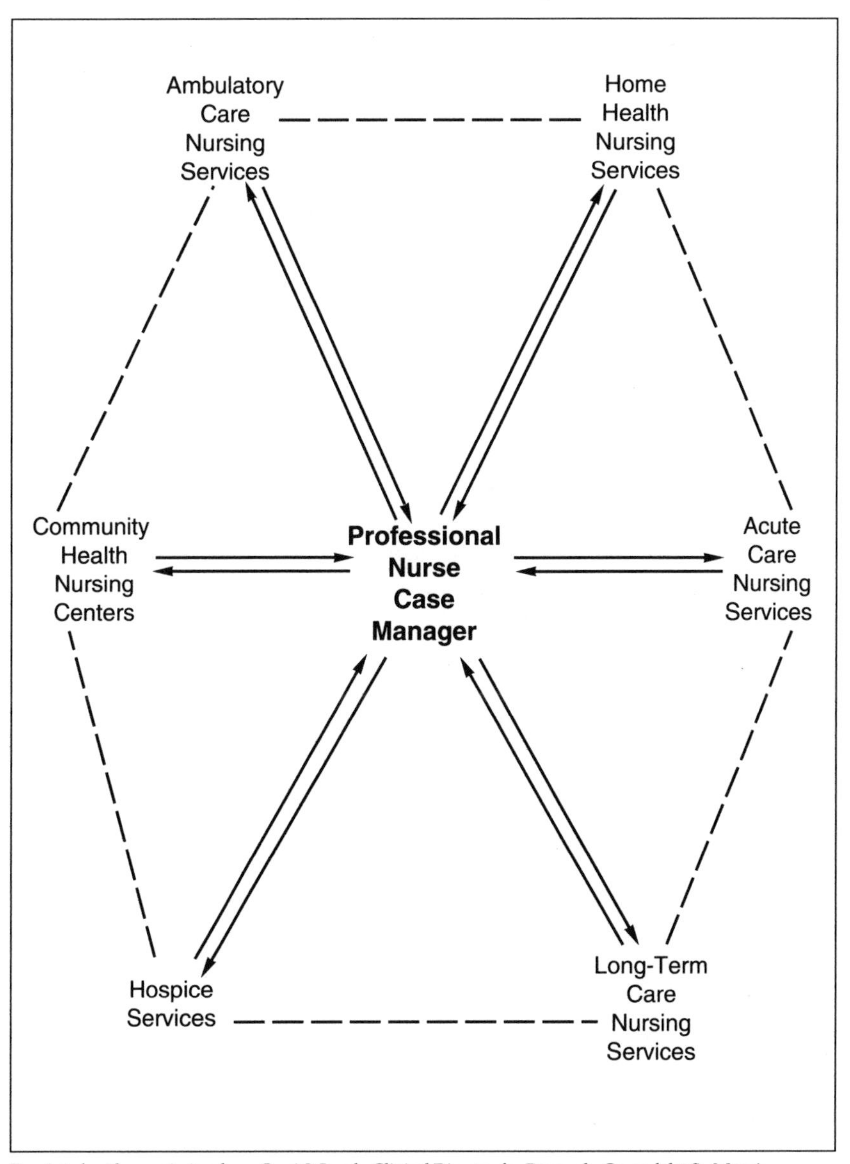

Reprinted with permission from Gerri S. Lamb, Clinical Director for Research, Carondelet St. Mary's Hospital and Health Center, Tucson, Arizona.

hold other positions and practice part-time in the nurse case manager role are prepared at the master's or doctoral level. The experience gained at Carondelet St. Mary's has demonstrated that working with clients over time to achieve targeted quality and cost outcomes requires experience and expertise in comprehensive health assessment, communication, advocacy, short- and long-term goal setting, service planning, and evaluation.

In 1990, the nursing case management experiences provided a foundation for beginning a hospital-based nursing health maintenance organization. Services within the capitated nursing HMO contract include nursing case management, Medicare home health services, infusion and in-home nursing care, and respite services to high-risk elderly clients enrolled in a medical HMO (Michaels, in press). The nurse case manager plays a pivotal role in this contract as a direct provider and in facilitating access to other nursing and health care services. The nurse case manager collaborates with the client, family, and other health professionals to design, implement, and evaluate the plans of care that are most suited to each individual's needs and goals. The volume and pace of services within the HMO have necessitated the use of laptop computers for documentation, as well as cellular telephones and voice mailboxes for communication.

During extensive interviews, clients who have received nursing case management were asked about their experiences. In these interviews, clients emphasized the significance of their relationship with the nurse case manager and the importance of the opportunity to voice their concerns to a caring, knowledgeable professional. Clients identified numerous outcomes that they associated with nursing case management, including improved coping and symptoms management, increased satisfaction with their health care, and changes in their use of health services, such as reduced reliance on the emergency department and longer spans between hospitalizations (Lamb and Stempel, 1991). Some client comments about nursing case management at Carondelet St. Mary's were:

- "You leave the security of the hospital where you have somebody watching you and taking care of you. And then, pretty soon, you are left alone and it's really hard" [it is at this point that the nurse case manager intervenes].
- "[The nurse case manager] helps me calm down and then I feel like I can handle it."

- "[The nurse case manager] gives me other avenues to think about."
- "Before I got hooked up with the nurse case manager, I was in the hospital every couple of months."

In comparison studies, individuals who received nursing case management were found to have shorter lengths of hospital stay, lower acuity at admission to the hospital, and fewer critical care days than individuals who did not receive nursing case management (Ethridge and Lamb, 1989; Chapman, 1990). Another study in progress at Carondelet St. Mary's is examining the impact of nursing case management on quality and cost outcomes for a younger population with the progressive chronic illness of multiple sclerosis.

Hennepin County Medical Center Model

Hennepin County Medical Center (HCMC) is a 520-bed public teaching hospital in Minneapolis. It is the only Level I Trauma Center in Minnesota. HCMC admits approximately 17,000 patients annually and operates one of the largest clinic systems in Minnesota.

At HCMC, case management is a client-centered, quality management program. It enhances the function of the health care team and increases their span of control over their practice. Case managers collaborate with physicians and ancillary departments to coordinate a course of treatment throughout the episode of care. Case management facilitators provide support to the case management system by assisting practitioners with the development, implementation, and evaluation of specific case type projects.

With the client at the center of the model, case management fosters quality of care by clearly identifying standards and outcomes for a case type. A feature of the HCMC program is the integration of case management into existing systems such as quality management, documentation, and nurse and physician orientation. Multidisciplinary and interdepartmental collaboration ensures that clients, families, and caregivers work together to achieve the desired care outcomes.

Since its introduction at HCMC, case management has been responsible for more than $1 million of direct cost savings. At the same time, significant improvement in quality of care has been demonstrated. The following case types exemplify improvements in effectiveness and efficiency at HCMC as a result of case management:

	Prior to Case Management	After Case Management
DRG 148 (Major small and large bowel procedures)		
• ICU length of stay	14 days	6 days
• Readmission rate	26%	6%
• Direct cost	$13,296	$12,167
DRG 210 (Hip and femur procedures except major joint, over 17 years old, with coexisting comorbidities)		
• Length of stay	12 days	8 days
• Compliance with antibiotic protocol	38%	89%
• Direct cost	$6,541	$4,173
DRG 014 (Specific cerebrovascular disorders, except transischemic attack)		
• Length of stay	10.2 days	6.97 days
• Readmission rate	43%	31%
• Direct cost	$3,501	$2,141

Medical University of South Carolina Medical Center Model

The Medical University of South Carolina (MUSC) Medical Center, located in Charleston, is a 557-bed teaching hospital with over 207,000 outpatient clinic visits annually. Nursing case management was implemented at MUSC in August 1988. The organizational structure of the nursing department consists of four clinical divisions (surgical, medical, cardiovascular, and maternal-infant), each with its own clinical director. The management team in each division consists of case managers who must be MSN-prepared and nurse managers who must be at least BSN-prepared. Both groups are aligned equally in the organizational structure. Typically, the case managers manage the patient care while the nurse managers manage the nursing staff.

At MUSC, case managers function in a variety of roles, including clinical expert, educator, manager, collaborator, and researcher. The primary responsibility of the case manager, however, is the management of the resources necessary and appropriate to achieve desired patient outcomes within a designated length of stay. In order to accomplish this, the case manager collaborates with the physicians, nurses, and ancillary departments involved in the patient's care. The case manager then coordinates the plan of care, the discharge plan, and the utilization of resources for the individual patient. The case manager serves as a resource in the identification of interdisciplinary interventions necessary to meet desired outcomes.

Upon admission, all patients are assigned to a case manager aligned with the specialty care need for which they are admitted. At MUSC, the case managers are service-/specialty-oriented, rather than unit-based. Therefore, a case manager may have patients located on many different units. The case manager follows patients from admission throughout the episode of illness, and makes community or home health referrals. Some case managers will continue contact with their patients during subsequent clinic visits.

The MUSC Medical Center Case Management Model was designed as an integrated system, and includes the components of standards of patient care, problem lists, and critical pathways. In this program, a list of priority problems is developed for each patient. Patient care is then guided and supported by the appropriate standards of patient care and the critical pathway. This process is reflected in Figure 2.

Depending on the case managers' individual nursing specialties, the patient populations of some case managers are more heavily concentrated in outpatient clinics rather than on inpatient units. While providing essential care for all patients, case managers also have developed individual practices to meet the unique needs of specialized patient populations. Some case managers are now beginning to focus primarily on the designated high-risk patients, continuing to serve as a resource for low-risk patients only as needs or problems arise.

The impact of case management on length of stay and the financial components of care at MUSC Medical Center is currently being assessed. The overall response to case management, however, has been extremely positive from all disciplines. The key characteristic of the MUSC program is that one person — the case manager — is thoroughly familiar with a patient and all aspects of the patient's care throughout the hospital stay and on subsequent admissions.

Figure 2
MUSC Medical Center
Case Management Model

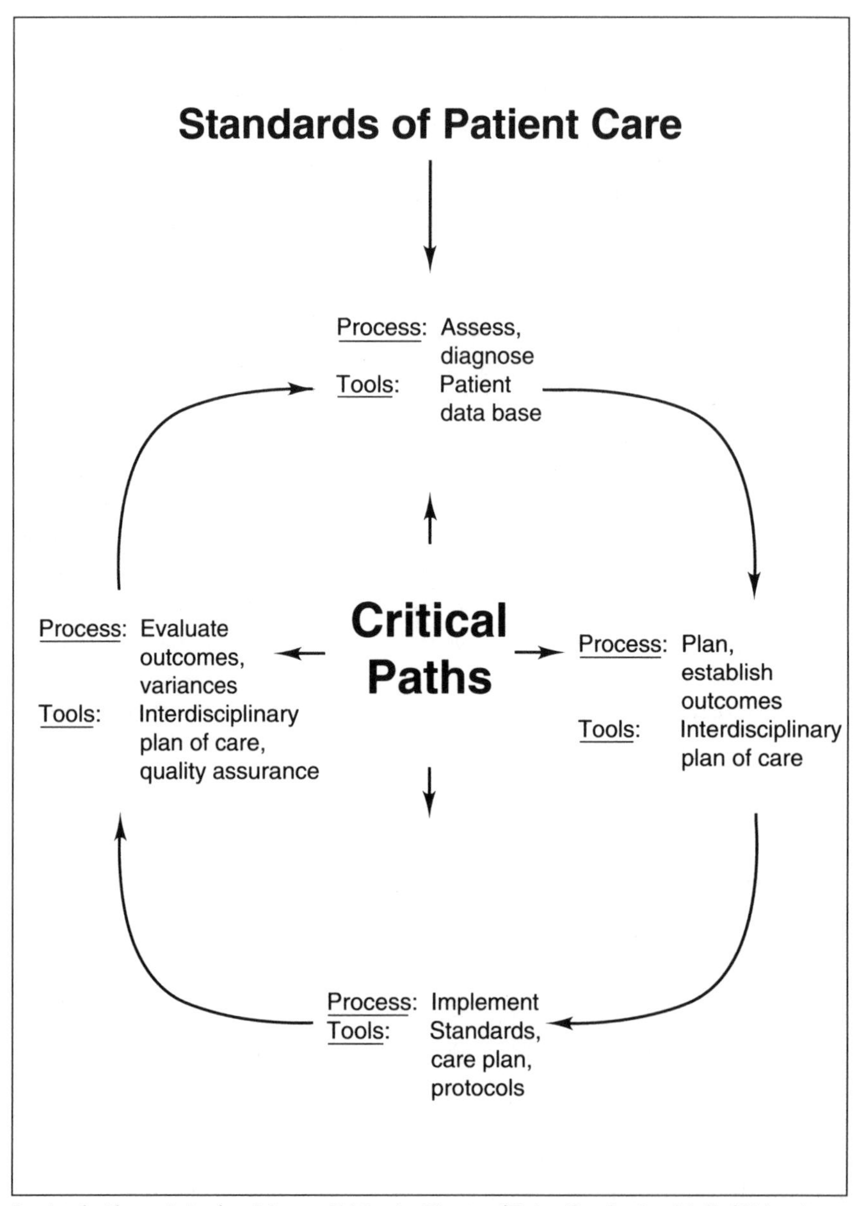

Reprinted with permission from Maureen K. Maguire, Director of Patient Care Services, Medical University of South Carolina, Charleston, South Carolina.

New Jersey Department of Health Model: Perinatal AIDS Prevention Project

The New Jersey Perinatal AIDS Prevention Project offers case management services to women who are either HIV-infected or at high risk for HIV infection in the cities of Newark, Jersey City, and Paterson. Services in these target cities are available at three types of sites. Prenatal clinics in each city provide case management services for women who are HIV-infected or at high risk for infection. Family planning clinics also provide services to this group, emphasizing risk reduction behavior. Citywide coordinators are also available to provide services to HIV-infected women in the community who are not seriously ill with the virus.

The New Jersey Perinatal AIDS Prevention Project has developed a case management system to ensure the provision of services to women who have the AIDS virus or HIV infection, or who are identified as being at high risk for contracting the infection. The ultimate goal of the project is to reduce the risk of transmission of the HIV infection by women of reproductive age.

The specific activities of the case manager in this project form the framework of the system:

- Psychosocial needs assessment.
- Medical needs and access to care.
- HIV risk assessment, knowledge, and education.
- Service plan development.
- Referral services.
- Individual and group counseling.
- Support groups.
- Intense follow-up.
- Reassessment of client needs for services.

Nursing case management services through the New Jersey Perinatal AIDS Prevention Project began in February 1990. To date, approximately 220 women are enrolled in the case management program. Results of the project's interventions will be available in 1992.

Nursing Center Model

Trimark Health Service, Inc. of Atlanta, Georgia, is an example of a community nursing organization that provides case management services within the community. Trimark is a strategic vehicle for achieving the objectives of case management and delivering high-quality, cost-effective health care.

Trimark provides services and products that enhance the physical and mental health or functional capacity of individuals within their homes or outside an institutional setting. The services provided include nursing visits and private duty care. Private duty care may be professional nursing care or personal care delivered by nursing assistants supervised by professional nurses.

The delivery of health care services at home has significantly increased in recent years. Factors influencing this growth include:

- Increasing consumer awareness and self-care.
- Technological advances.
- Demographic changes.
- Increased competition in the health care marketplace.
- Payment systems that encourage shortened hospital lengths of stay.

Health care at home is one of the competitive options for cost-effective health care. Price competition combined with quality services delivered in the home environment (usually far more desirable than an institutional setting when institutional care is not essential) makes home health care an attractive option.

Trimark works with various case management networks, including case management companies, insurers, self-insured employers, managed care systems (health maintenance organizations and preferred provider operations), and other health care providers. Case managers refer clients to Trimark as an alternative to extended hospitalization or admission to other long-term care settings. Individuals who are expected to be dependent on nursing care for an extended period of time, such as technology-dependent clients, may be referred to Trimark for around-the-clock nursing care.

The utilization controls inherent in case management provided through managed care systems encourage the use of care at home to shorten hospital lengths of stay. Many clients and families are taught self-care in the home. For example, clients in the home may receive total parenteral nutrition, infusion for antibiotic therapy, pain control, cancer chemotherapy, and phototherapy. Case management inherently assumes a close working relationship between the case manager and the provider.

Trimark also provides case management within the community at large. Because of his or her position in the continuum of services, the Trimark nurse can identify the needs of clients requiring case management, develop a plan of care, and refer clients to other appropriate services as needed. Trimark provides the nursing and personal care services as defined by the case management plan.

In one example of case management by Trimark, the nurse works with residents in a retirement community. When the nurse identifies that a resident is having difficultly maintaining personal hygiene and grooming, a condition which may threaten his or her ability to live in the retirement community, the case management plan is begun. The nurse as case manager works with the resident to provide personal care services and to determine whether a health problem is causing the client's lapse in personal hygiene. In some instances, referral to a physician or other health care service is indicated. Family and retirement community management are included in the case management process as appropriate.

Trimark may provide some or all of the hands-on care that the client requires within the case management plan, such as health education, the adaptation of life-style to disease limitations, family support and teaching, identification of and referral to community resources, nursing services, and personal care services.

Another focus for case management is eldercare, a program that addresses the problems of middle-aged adults who have responsibility for the care of elderly relatives. Responsibility for this care most often falls to a daughter or daughter-in-law of an elderly parent. Because of the increasing number of women in the work force, those who have eldercare responsibilities are losing time away from their jobs. This situation is attracting the attention of major businesses and industries. Services targeted to large employers and the middle-aged population can significantly reduce the pressures of eldercare.

Case management, including respite care and direct personal care, is the core component of Trimark's eldercare program. The nurse as case manager evaluates the client's needs and determines appropriate referral sources. When Trimark provides eldercare case management, it plans and coordinates services based on the changing needs of the older person and family. Among the services to be coordinated, along with nursing and personal care, are meals-on-wheels, selection of health care providers, adult day care, evaluation of housing options, and consideration of nursing home placement.

Charges for case management of home health services are incorporated within the charge for nursing and personal care services. Separate charges may also be made for specific case management services. Payment sources include direct out-of-pocket payment and third-party reimbursement through insurance or managed care payers. Medicaid pays for services resulting from case management in some states. Medicare does not pay for case management per se.

Case management services are provided for those clients who have ongoing or periodic health care needs. Those clients in the home health environment who most frequently need case management are those with chronic or terminal illness and the elderly.

Health Maintenance Organization Model

Prime Health, a staff-model health maintenance organization based in Kansas City, Missouri, uses a case management program. Prime Health has 66,000 members, approximately 3,000 of whom require case management services due to the complexity of their care as inpatients, referred clients, and/or home care clients (Prime Health, 1987).

The first case management services offered by Prime Health were provided by Care Options, Inc., which was created by a nurse. Prime Health contracted with Care Options for case management services provided by nurses, wherein the primary care physician, the nurse, and the client acted as a team. The nurse case manager was given responsibility for utilization review, quality assurance, and individual case management.

This dimension of service, which has been integrated into the total program, has undergone several organizational changes and is now known as the Case Management Division of Prime Health, Kansas City.

The vice president for case management, a registered nurse prepared at the doctoral level, is responsible for administering the program. The Kansas City staff consists of eight baccalaureate- and master's-prepared nurses. Prime Health has a management contract with a university-based HMO in Mobile, Alabama. The Case Management Division, Kansas City, is responsible for administering, staffing, and directing case management at the Mobile HMO. Three nurses are located at the Mobile site.

According to the formal mission statement of Prime Health (Prime Health, 1987), the goal of case management is "to facilitate the delivery of optimum quality health care in the most cost-effective manner through collaboration with health teams, professionals, community agencies, Prime Health administration, and Prime Health members."

The mission statement also outlines the following objectives for case management at Prime Health:

- Monitor all inpatient, referral, and home health services according to established criteria.
- Interpret benefit coverage to physicians, other health care providers, and members.
- Serve as a resource for providers regarding appropriate and alternative delivery settings, systems, and interventions.
- Collaborate with primary care providers in developing and implementing risk management programs for care delivered to members in episodic, ambulatory, and community settings.
- Challenge the status quo in the interest of improving productivity, quality, and creativity within the Prime Health delivery system.

The nurse case manager is responsible for preadmission certification, admission, and concurrent review. The nurse case manager interacts with providers and clients prior to, during, and following hospitalization. This interaction includes assessment, education, planning, appropriate direct care, evaluation, and feedback. The nurse case manager conducts a retrospective analysis of data, including non-acute profile studies, and engages in quality assurance and utilization review activities. Additional responsibilities of the nurse case manager include research and development of new policies, procedures, standards, and treatment of modalities. A nurse case manager is available to Prime Health 24 hours-a-day, seven days-a-week.

The role of the nurse case manager at Prime Health is unique in that his or her responsibilities span the entire organizational structure and include administrative as well as clinical responsibilities.

Public Health Model

In New Jersey, the Gloucester County Health Department uses case management methodology to promote early identification, evaluation, diagnosis, and treatment of children with special health needs and potentially handicapping conditions. Because of the success of the Gloucester County program, community-based case management units have been developed in a statewide program.

Local case management units serve as entry points into the health care system to provide coordinated and comprehensive care for children under 21 years of age who may have special health needs as the result of a disease, defect, or condition that may hinder normal growth and development. Collaboration and networking with existing local and regional agencies serving the needs of handicapped children facilitate this process. The case manager, a nurse, works actively with child and parent to coordinate services and is responsible for the following:

- Counseling the parent and child regarding problem identification, and validating their level of knowledge and understanding.
- Assessing the needs for services, and developing with the parent an individualized service plan that addresses medical, education, developmental, social, and rehabilitative needs.
- Assisting the child and parent to reach the goals identified in the service plan by taking an active part in the procurement of services from appropriate community agencies.
- Being available to the family as a resource in crisis, responding actively to complaints about services, and providing objective information about alternatives for securing direct services.
- Promoting and facilitating communication among providers serving the child and parent.
- Monitoring the services received by the child and family by reviewing the receipt of services and the child's progress toward the attainment of goals identified in the service plan.

The case manager is a public health nurse with at least two years of experience in pediatrics. The recommended caseload is approximately 300 to 350 children per case manager. In units with very large caseloads, interdisciplinary teams include master's-prepared social workers with two years of experience in working with handicapped children and families. All cases are monitored on a systematic basis, depending on the needs of the client and family and the severity of the handicap.

Case management services are available through contract funding from the New Jersey State Department of Health and are supplemented by local county revenues. Services are voluntary and available to all county residents (New Jersey State Department of Health, 1983).

Through expansion in the development of model waiver programs, New Jersey now provides direct reimbursement to county units for case management services to children whose health care is less expensive in the home setting than it would be in the hospital or extended care facility.

Acute Care Model

Nursing case management in the hospital setting is in the hands of primary nurses at the New England Medical Center in Boston. Case management is client-centered and emphasizes client outcomes and individual nurse accountability.

Prior to an individual's hospitalization, a nurse case manager contacts the individual at home to provide an orientation to care. At this time, the nurse identifies other health problems that might compromise recovery and necessitate individualization of the established protocols (mutually set by nurse and physician) to determine the critical path of the case management plan.

A critical path identifies predictable, critical, or key incidents which must occur at set times to achieve an appropriate length of stay in the hospital. For example, an individual recuperating from a myocardial infarction typically could be expected to be out of the bed to a chair on the third day of hospitalization, and ambulatory in the room on the fifth day.

By the time the client is admitted, the case manager is able to describe the critical path of the client's stay, the unit where the client will be housed before surgery, the name of the primary nurse on that unit, and procedures that will take place. The individual will be told the name of the primary nurse on each unit where he or she will reside, and the events that will occur each day (e.g., catheter removal, discontinuation of intravenous fluids, first meal tray, and visiting regulations).

During hospitalization, the individual's progress along the critical path is evaluated every eight hours, and adjustments are made as necessary in the care plan. The critical path tracks health outcomes, nurse-dependent complications, activity outcomes, and knowledge outcomes.

The nurse case manager is the primary nurse for the client in the unit where the individual will be housed during hospitalization, and monitors the client's progress and advocates for the client throughout the entire hospitalization. Discharge planning is outlined before admission and completed by the time of discharge. Thereafter, the nurse case manager is available to the client by phone for information or reassurance, and becomes the nurse case manager for the individual on subsequent admissions. A primary nurse is case manager for 15–20 hospitalized clients.

At the New England Medical Center, cost and length of stay are two outcomes of case management. Case managers have a projected cost (resource) and length of stay (budget) for each case. The standardized budgets permit evaluation of the success of nurse case managers in reaching outcomes according to the time line. Typical problem-oriented quality assurance programs are used to evaluate the quality of care.

A four-part audit also is conducted every four months on the work of every primary nurse. These audits include a self-audit, a peer chart audit, a client/family audit (interview), and a unit leadership (vertical) audit. A second approach to evaluating the quality of care is the outcome audit, whereby achievement of predetermined outcomes and intermediate goals is evaluated. Evaluation can be accomplished by observing and interviewing the client and family, or auditing closed records. As outcomes are derived from nursing standards, analysis of the outcomes gives an evaluation of the quality of care.

Concurrent audits also offer information on cost. The audits permit rapid revisions in care based on changes in the client's condition. Therefore, the costs are revealed in relation to actual interventions and their anticipated versus actual outcomes. As explained by Zander (1988c), when case-based financial reports are available to key clinicians, "the interdependencies between cost and quality can be better understood and managed." Nursing case management produces a more accurate account of true costs of acute care, because tasks and interventions are in a cause-effect relationship with outcomes occurring within time frames.

Hospital-Based Models for Persons with AIDS

San Francisco General Hospital

The use of case management in treating persons with acquired immune deficiency syndrome (AIDS) has been highly successful in San Francisco. As Figure 3 indicates, the case management system

Figure 3
Public Health and AIDS

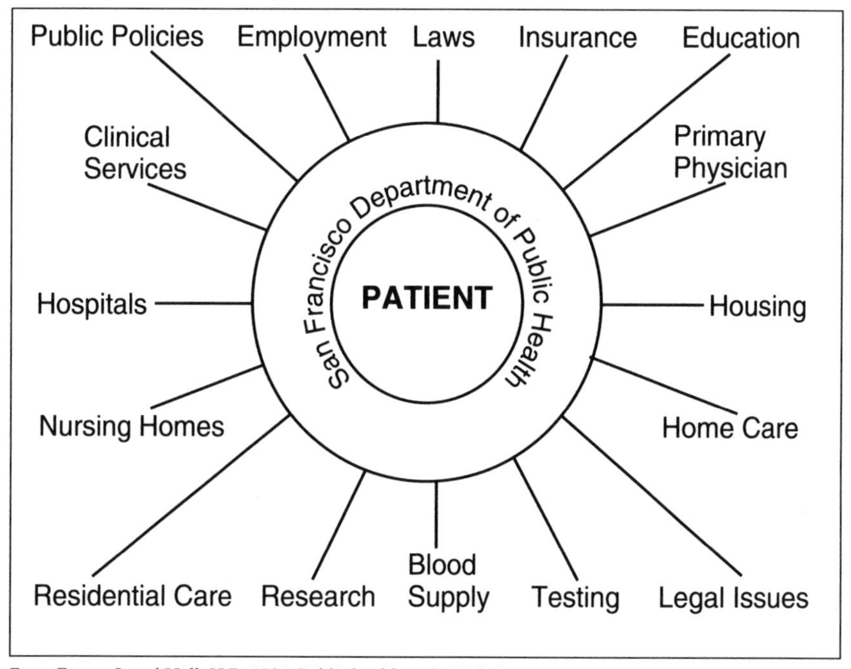

From Foster, J. and Hall, H.D. 1986. Public health and AIDS. *Caring* 5(6):4. Reprinted with permission by the National Association for Home Care, Washington, D.C.

pioneered at San Francisco General Hospital follows the public health model, minimizing the time clients spend in the hospital, stressing outpatient services, and creating a strong network of community support ranging from home care to hospice to housing. This model of care focuses on the development of out-of-hospital services to reduce dependency on more expensive and often unnecessary hospitalizations.

Indicators of success for the San Francisco model of care include the following:

- The community support system enhances the quality of life for persons with AIDS.
- Because case management results in shorter lengths of stay in hospitals, the average length of stay at San Francisco General Hospital is 11 days — compared to a national average of 19 days.
- In San Francisco, persons with AIDS receive treatment for approximately half the cost of such services in other cities.
- The outpatient AIDS clinic at San Francisco General Hospital averages about 1,600 visits per month; the inpatient unit has the capacity for 20 clients; and an overflow of 20 or more clients are placed throughout the hospital.
- Whether a person with AIDS enters the system for care through San Francisco General Hospital or requests the services of one of the community-based agencies, he or she automatically gains access to the case management system, since all the institutions and agencies are linked together through the coordinating efforts of the AIDS Office of the San Francisco Department of Public Health.
- Medi-Cal, California's Medicaid system, has cooperated with local and state agencies. People with AIDS now automatically become eligible for Medi-Cal benefits, making it much easier to establish a continuum of services.

Some background on the groups, institutions, and agencies serving persons with AIDS in San Francisco will illustrate the city's commitment to helping these persons and preventing the spread of the disease.

The gay community, the group most affected by AIDS in San Francisco, was well-organized and established at the outbreak of the epidemic. The San Francisco Department of Public Health used its long-standing relationship with the gay community to plan and develop services.

The department provided leadership and acted swiftly early in the epidemic. An AIDS office was established within the department and an AIDS coordinating committee was appointed to organize and establish monitoring mechanisms for organizations involved in the prevention, health education, and housing needs of persons with AIDS, as well as in providing home, community-based, and hospice care services required by persons with AIDS.

At San Francisco General Hospital , an AIDS clinic was established in January 1983. A clinical nurse specialist was appointed as clinical AIDS coordinator for inpatient services, and an inpatient unit was established by July 1983. With the merging of outpatient and inpatient services into a coordinated system, case management for persons with AIDS was initiated. Both outpatient and inpatient services sought support from community groups and included them in planning and decision making as the program developed, thereby eliciting their cooperation.

The inpatient program, designed by nurses, is a nurse-run unit using a modified primary nursing model with an all-RN staff. The client is the center of care. This nursing model is effective because AIDS is a nursing-oriented disease, requiring the nurse's clinical, psychosocial, and collaborative skills.

A clinical nurse specialist and a social worker are responsible for case management and coordinate the discharge planning process, a primary focus for inpatient services. The client collaborates in establishing his or her plan — outlining the critical path he or she will follow. Extensive networking occurs among professionals and community supporters to assure that when clients with AIDS are ready to leave the hospital, they have a place to go and have the care and support they need.

The San Francisco AIDS Foundation, the Shanti Project, and the Visiting Nurses Association play key roles in meeting the needs of persons with AIDS. The San Francisco AIDS Foundation provides information, education, and prevention services. The foundation serves as an advocacy, social services, and referral agency, in addition to operating a food bank for persons diagnosed with AIDS.

The Shanti Project, established in 1974 before the AIDS epidemic, provides volunteer support for persons with life-threatening illnesses and offers assistance to persons with AIDS. The project provides 1) volunteer emotional support services; 2) practical support services that include housekeeping chores, shopping, errands, and transportation; and 3) a residential housing component that utilizes multi-bedroom residences for shared housing of people with common problems.

The Visiting Nurse Association's home care and hospice team provides comprehensive home care and hospice services, and staffs a residential inpatient hospice — Coming Home Hospice — in the convent of a Catholic parish.

If a person is seen by a private physician or is treated at a private hospital (two-thirds of the persons with AIDS in San Francisco now receive care in the private sector), he or she can still access the services of the community-based agencies. Most of the private institutions and physicians in San Francisco recognize the value of these services and have developed formal or informal relationships with these agencies. Once a patient has gained access to the case management system, he or she may use any of the services as needed.

The City of San Francisco has financed the development of the AIDS program at San Francisco General Hospital, and has contracts with each of the community-based agencies to provide services. This has allowed the city to develop the most comprehensive continuum of services for persons with AIDS, at the lowest cost, of any city in the country (Genna, 1987).

Articles describing the San Francisco services in greater detail include "Public Health and AIDS" (Foster and Hall, 1986), "AIDS Management" (Genna, 1987), and "Establishing a Therapeutic Environment: Institutional Resources" (Morrison, 1987).

St. Clare's Hospital, New York, New York

St. Clare's Hospital and Medical Center in New York is a 250-bed Roman Catholic institution located on Manhattan's West Side. St. Clare's operates under the auspices of the Archdiocese of New York, and is affiliated with New York Medical College. St. Clare's has established the East Coast's largest dedicated unit for clients with AIDS.

The program has 60 acute-care inpatient beds, 10 of which are in a secured section for prisoners from the New York State correctional system. The program is staffed entirely by those who have chosen to work with persons with AIDS.

Genna (1987) notes that the outpatient service, which began in January 1986, has about 600 visits per month from some 800 registered clients. It offers screening for infection from the human immune deficiency virus (HIV), diagnostic and treatment services, AZT therapy, an ambulatory infusion program, extensive psychosocial programs, and a screening clinic. There is also a dental program for people who are HIV-positive. The program operates a toll-free national hotline that averages approximately 1,000 calls per week.

St. Clare's has developed a network with linkages to community-based services. The case management model used at St. Clare's was developed for a comprehensive AIDS program based at one facility. The person with HIV infection receives nursing, medical, social, pastoral, nutritional, psychiatric, outpatient, and housing services.

A case management team with representatives from various disciplines meets regularly to review clients and maintain continuity of care for case management aspects ranging from medical services to discharge planning. Community affiliations include a contract with the Visiting Nurses Association of New York to provide home care, and affiliations with two residences to provide housing for homeless persons. Volunteer services are provided by the hospital's volunteer program and by the Gay Men's Health Crisis, which operates a buddy system to provide emotional and practical support to a large number of persons with HIV infection. St. Clare's was involved in establishing and developing the New York City AIDS Service Delivery Consortium, and remains a member of this group, which integrates state and city agencies and many of the community-based organizations in New York City.

Genna (1987) reports that the client population at St. Clare's is composed of about 55 percent intravenous drug users and 45 percent homosexual/bisexual men. Sixty percent of the clients are from minority groups, a reflection of New York's demographics. Minorities often do not access the system until relatively late in their illness. The intravenous drug user tends to develop pneumocystis carinii pneumonia; therefore, his or her average length of stay is longer than that of others. The psychosocial needs of persons with AIDS are often great, their home situations are likely to be unstable, and finding them housing tends to be a great problem. The overall management of these clients is often complicated; therefore, their hospital stays tend to be lengthy.

Housing is a citywide problem in New York, and St. Clare's residence affiliations provide for only a fraction of the housing needed by the clients. The hospital is planning a 20-bed residence for homeless people and a 33-bed neuropsychiatric unit for persons with dementia and other neurological conditions caused by HIV infection. Plans also include expansion of the prison unit to 25 beds, and establishment of a methadone maintenance treatment program for persons with HIV infection.

Financing for this model comes from a variety of sources. St. Clare's was officially designated as the first AIDS center by the New York State Department of Health in February 1986. This made the hospital eligible for an enhanced Medicaid reimbursement rate for AIDS patients. The hospital receives $550 a day for inpatients and $55 for each outpatient visit. It has a low capital debt and a small physician training program, both enhancing the institution's ability to care for rsons with AIDS in a cost-effective manner.

Third-Party Payer Case Management Model

Virtually every major private insurer in the U.S. offers case management services. From a historical perspective, Liberty Mutual, headquartered in Boston, is most widely credited with implementing the first insurance-based program to apply case management practices to the medical field.

Liberty Mutual used medical management principles for over 30 years in workers' compensation cases to assist injured workers to return to work. Then, after reviewing claims data, the group health insurance industry identified that 80 percent of the total health care costs were incurred by 20 percent of the insured clients.

As they continued to evaluate the data, Liberty Mutual identified cases to be catastrophic by diagnosis. They also included those chronic diagnoses expected to involve high-dollar costs over a long term.

Patient conditions considered catastrophic and chronic that commonly receive case management services include:

- High-risk neonatal
- Severe head trauma
- Spinal cord injury
- Ventilator dependency
- Coma
- Multiple fractures
- AIDS
- Severe burns
- Cerebral vascular accidents
- Amputations
- Terminal illnesses
- Substance abuse

For the private payer, case managers focus on patients/clients with chronic and catastrophic injuries and illnesses considered high cost cases. Case managers coordinate all parties involved to maximize health care benefits and the quality of patient care (see Figure 4). Case management has been accepted by third-party payers because the care for the severely ill or injured often is excessively expensive due to lack of coordination, failure to know about and use lower-cost alternatives to hospital care, and duplication and fragmentation of services.

The process of case management includes:

- Case identification and referral. Patients are usually referred as early as possible after being screened according to diagnostic, clinical, and cost criteria. Only a small number of cases are referrals. Contact with a case manager may be initiated by the insurance company, the employer, the physician, and/or the patient/family.
- Case screening. The patient's medical and psychosocial needs are assessed and evaluated by telephone or an on-site visit. The patient's medical records and claims history are reviewed. The case manager seeks to identify short- and long-range treatment needs of the patient from the attending physician.
- Case implementation. The case manager sets up a network of communication between the patient, physicians, and any health care providers involved. Alternatives are evaluated, insurance benefits are defined, and all parties agree to a plan. The case manager presents the plan, which takes advantage of cost-effective alternatives and ensures quality patient care, to the payer.
- Case monitoring. The case manager monitors the plan and has regular contact with all parties involved.
- Case closure. The case manager remains involved until the highest level of functional health is achieved by the patient or closure criteria are achieved (i.e., patient dies, or insurance coverage is exhausted).

Third-party payers focus on containing costs, although all case management programs have as an equally important goal quality medical care and improvement of patient and family life. Case managers are now acting as patient advocates and liaisons between the patient and all parties involved to develop appropriate, cost-effective

Figure 4
Third-Party Payer Case Management Model

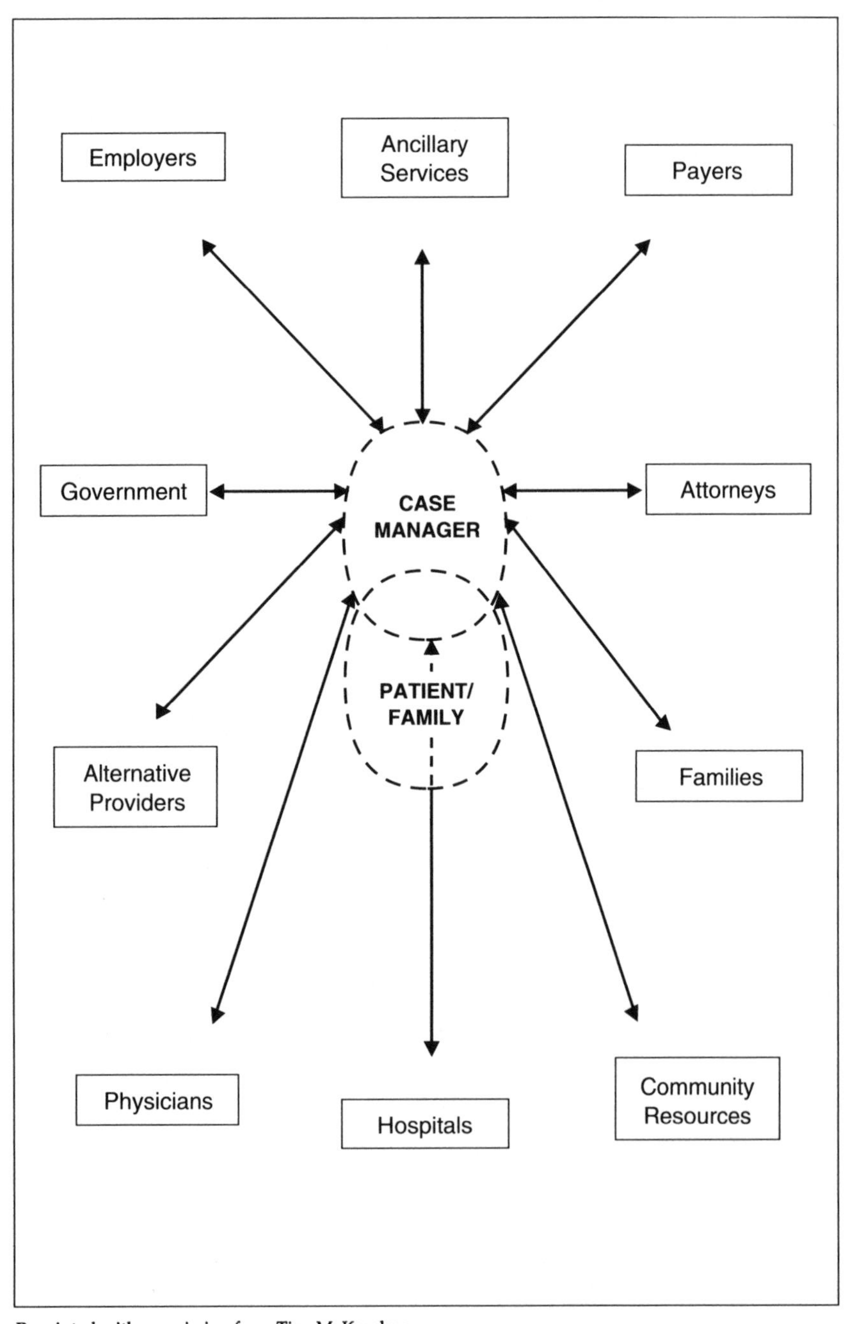

Reprinted with permission from Tina M. Kowlsen

health care plans. Using their clinical expertise and good communication skills, case managers can influence the kind and amount of services provided, and the order in which they are rendered, to achieve optimum efficiency.

A good working relationship between the physician and the case manager is critical. Case managers do not attempt to usurp the role of the physician. Physician cooperation and acceptance of case management services is essential, since the physician serves as the primary source of information in determining the patient's treatment plan. The physician strongly influences the patient's acceptance of case management services. All health care services still must be ordered through the physician.

The effects of case management services are important to third-party payers. Reports evaluating the process and outcome are requested more frequently. Standards for measuring the quality of the case management process and its effect on patient and payer outcomes are still evolving.

Most third-party payers use registered nurses with five years or more of clinical experience as case managers. Some programs are staffed by other types of health care professionals, such as rehabilitation counselors or social workers. Case managers working with or for third-party payers often interface with case managers in other programs. Coordination of services is essential to avoid duplication of efforts.

Caseloads vary from company to company, with an average of 16–20 cases per case manager. Case coordination becomes important since many cases are active at one time, although some cases may require less monitoring than others. Some companies provide only telephone case management services, and contract with independent case managers for on-site services. Other companies may provide both telephone and on-site services.

Ultimately, case management strives to maximize a patient's health and benefits through timely coordination of health care services. The quality of patient and family life requires interdisciplinary cooperation and coordination.

Case Management in Head Injury Rehabilitation*

Head injury rehabilitation lends itself quite naturally to a systems-based case management model because of the wide variety of factors such rehabilitation encompasses. The historical and contemporary focus of rehabilitation continues to be on comprehensive, integrated, holistic care. Head injury sequelae cut across all levels of human functioning.

Systems-Focused Rehabilitation Model

The framework focuses on 1) the understanding of the disease across physiologic and psychosocial dimensions, 2) mutual goal setting and care planning, and 3) the discovery of patterns of functionality that emerge in the real-world context.

A rehabilitation model based on this philosophical framework focuses on collaborative practice networks, interdisciplinary or transdisciplinary functions, and overlapping areas of resource allocation and use. This approach is best applied in clinical conditions, such as traumatic brain injury, where the injury is diffuse and dynamic, treatment strategies are still in development, and prognostication and prediction of recovery is tentative.

Systems-Based Case Management

To help determine scope and function, Zander (1988b) points out that case management is both a model and a technology. Davis Cosgrove, president of Upjohn Healthcare Service in 1988, viewed case management as a problem-solving approach which promotes continuity of care and effective appropriation of services (Zander, 1988a). Thus, case management in its broadest scope serves to coordinate and integrate services, resources, communication, and expectations among the patient, family, treatment team, and payer (Ballew and Mink, 1986; Zander, 1988c). This coordination and integration is carried out through planning, organizing, implementing, and evaluating (Ballew and Mink, 1986). The following is a list of the major operational principles of a systems-based case management model:

- Overall functional performance is greater than the sum of the individual performance of separate tasks. For example, successful performance of the prerequisite motor and cog-

*From Whitman, M. 1991. Case management in head injury rehabilitation. *Rehabilitation Nursing* 16(1):19-22. Reprinted with permission by the Association of Rehabilitation Nurses, Skokie, Ill.

nitive tasks necessary for walking does not guarantee that the patient will functionally ambulate.

- Overall functional performance is more dependent on interactions than on actions. Therefore, the patient's ability to walk depends on an interaction among motor, cognitive, and other related skills.
- Disabilities, impairments, and handicaps really are systems of problems. Functional ambulation implies more than a means of walking. The patient must have sufficient intent, motivation, and purpose if he or she is to perform the task successfully.
- Optimum rehabilitation efforts are more than the sum of the optimal interventions used to remedy specific deficits. Each patient, family member, and staff member has a set of assumptions and expectations about the value of walking. Hence, optimum rehabilitation efforts must move beyond pure remediation of deficits toward providing all players with a common understanding of the significance of performing the task of walking.
- All elements in the rehabilitation process must be anticipated and planned for simultaneously and interdependently. A total rehabilitation plan must take into account the fact that ambulation occurs in diverse contexts, times, places, and conditions. Walking across the living room is not the same as walking across a busy city street at the height of rush hour.

A systems-based conceptual model for case management keeps us mindful that communication, expectations, resources, and services occur within clinical, rehabilitation, lifelong care, and patient/family subsystems (see Figure 5). Each of these subsystems exerts an influence on planning, organizing, implementing, and evaluating activities. These subsystems may try to steer the rehabilitation process in different directions; the case management model strives to integrate all of these influences and make the process move in a single direction.

Focus on Outcome: Planning, Organizing, Implementing, and Evaluating in Case Management

Planning. Case management planning begins by determining the ultimate discharge disposition. All further rehabilitation program-

Figure 5

Systems-Based Conceptual Model for Case Management Services

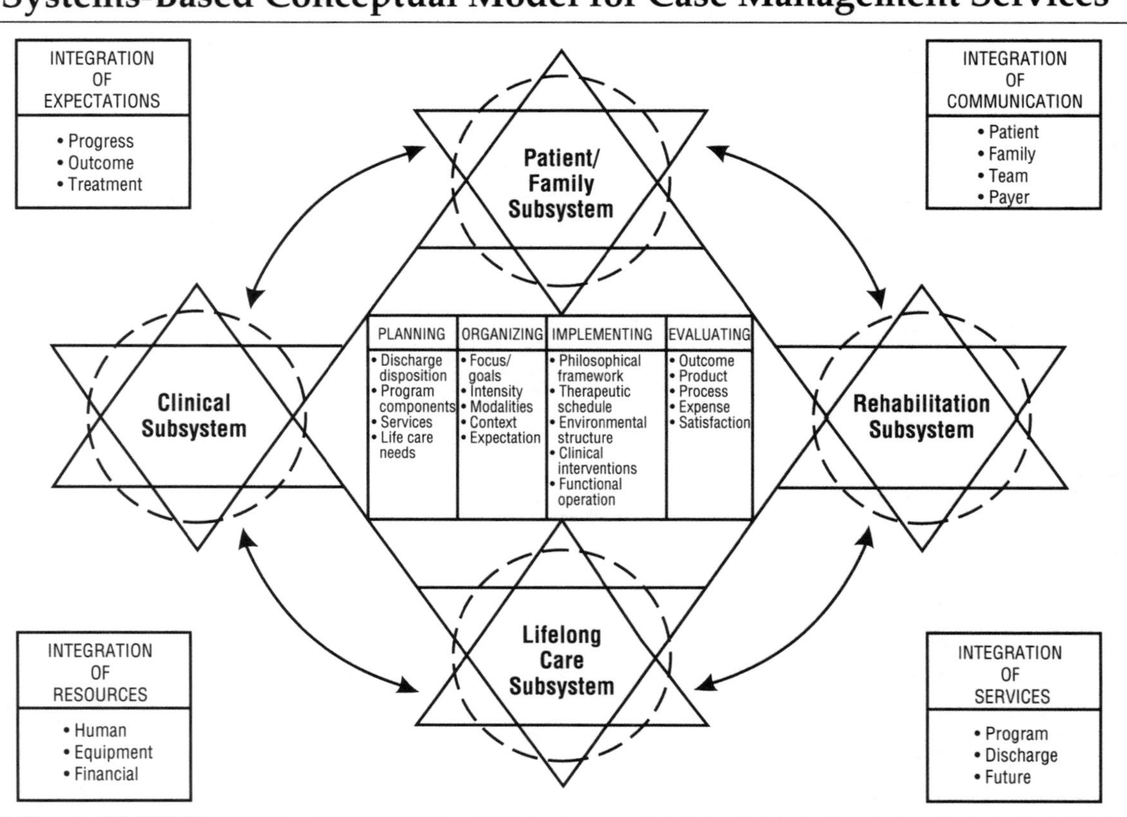

Reprinted with permission from the Association of Rehabilitation Nurses, Skokie, Ill.

ming and service delivery is built around this pivotal point. Contrary to the more common approach, which focuses on determining the patient's deficits and the treatment necessary to remediate those deficits, this focus first ascertains the targeted discharge site and then what absolutely must happen for this targeted discharge option to become a workable reality.

While this may seem a trivial theoretical distinction, the pragmatic differences actually are critical. The first approach may lead to compartmentalization of the patient and care; the second approach synthesizes a variety of perspectives and aims to identify essential barriers, consolidate rehabilitation efforts, and realize achievable outcomes. In the second approach, planning simultaneously weighs immediate, intermediate, and lifelong care needs to determine the focus and goals of treatment.

Organizing. Having identified the overall focus and goal of the patient's program, the next step is to develop a blueprint for how these goals will be met. This involves specifying the actual intensity, type, mix, and expectations of treatment methods and approaches. Several questions need to be addressed in the process:

- What are the primary areas of concentration?
- Which disciplines need to be involved in which areas, and to what extent?
- What areas need zones of overlapping treatment across disciplines?
- How will the patient's typical performance across tasks, functional areas, and time be measured, and by whom?
- How will factors such as poor concentration, tendency toward distraction, fatigue, and agitation influence the intensity, frequency, and duration of treatment?
- Which treatment modalities will best assure generalization of performance across tasks and environments?
- How do the patient's and family's expectations influence treatment opinions?

Considerable interdisciplinary involvement, coordination, and discussion are necessary to achieve consensus regarding answers to these questions, as well as to set the final direction for the patient's individualized treatment schedule and care plan.

Implementing. Program design and treatment always occur within a particular philosophical framework, organizational climate, and environment. Effective programming requires the creation and promotion of environments and perspectives conducive to recovery. Successful program implementation is strongly influenced by environmental factors and by staff, family, and patient attitudes. The philosophy of treatment must be sensitive to the traumatic brain injury patient's unique characteristics. Careful attention is needed to assure that cognitive and behavioral sequelae are interpreted and treated correctly. For example, incorrectly attributing cognitive deficits to motivational problems and behavioral deficits to manipulation can severely misdirect treatment efforts.

Environmental needs — such as distraction-free treatment areas, time-out rooms, and noninvasive security systems — play an important role in optimal treatment design. Other factors crucial in program implementation are availability of community-based treatment options and a flexible treatment approach that allows for skill performance in the real-world context. Three essential questions should be addressed during implementation:

1. Does the treatment design aim toward ever-increasing approximations of the real-world context?
2. Are functionally-relevant tasks presented in functionally-relevant ways so as to promote meaningful outcomes?
3. Can the successful performance seen in the rehabilitation environment be replicated and maintained in the real world?

Successful program evaluation is strongly dependent on affirmative responses to these questions.

Evaluating. Measuring and analyzing outcomes in head injury rehabilitation is fraught with difficulties. Some fairly common difficulties occur in differentiating 1) practice effects from consolidated gains, 2) spontaneous recovery from treatment-related recovery, and 3) meaningful function outcome from isolated progress in functional areas (Dikmen and Temkin, 1987; Diller and Ben-Yishay, 1987). Nonetheless, case management accountability requires developing a workable evaluation plan in the face of these problems.

To be useful, an evaluation approach must be capable of describing, tracking, and evaluating results throughout the dimensions of outcome, product, process, expense, and satisfaction. An outcome evaluation model that measures progress across the areas of pathology, impairment, disability, handicap, and environment can provide the type of comprehensive framework needed to capture salient improvements in this patient population. However, consideration must be given to both the product and the process by which gains are achieved and maintained. In the face of relevant functional improvement, one must ask what human, equipment, and environmental resources are required to support this level of functional performance, and at what expense.

The rehabilitation nurse's awareness of the impact of the subsystems on the rehabilitation process will enhance the nurse's ability to plan, organize, implement, and evaluate patient care. Comprehensive nursing observation occurs across all shifts and throughout the patient's stay. More than any other member of the rehabilitation team, the rehabilitation nurse has the skill and the long-term opportunity to assess a patient's progress. Therefore, the rehabilitation nurse is best equipped to assess the impact of subsystems on the rehabilitation program, and to ultimately affect the patient's outcome. This holistic nursing assessment establishes the foundation for a systems-based case management approach to care.

Orchestration of a systems-based case management model requires tremendous organizational and clinical commitment. Cost-effective programming relies heavily on the rehabilitation team's ability and willingness to target and address only the essential barriers to discharge placement — across disciplines and in a tightly integrated manner.

Consistency, continuity, and communication of shared expectations among the patient, family, health care team, and payer are essential if real-world outcomes are to have functional integrity and long-standing duration. Practically speaking, this is possible only in an environment where compassion becomes embodied in quality care.

Independent Geriatric Case Management Model

Community Care Consultants of Southfield, Michigan is an example of a nurse-owned organization that provides independent geriatric case management services within the community on a fee-for-service basis.

Community Care Consultants utilizes a functional model, rather than a model based on illness and disease, through which to provide independent geriatric case management services to older persons and their families. The organization provides services designed to maximize the potential of older persons and their families without disrupting life-styles, and to enhance the quality of life for the concerned family and older adult.

Nurses who provide independent geriatric case management possess a master's degree in nursing and have advanced preparation in gerontology. Advanced preparation is essential because of the complex care needs of older adults and their families, and the degree of difficulty in working with the components of the nursing process. For example, there is an enormous leap from multidimensional assessment to problem identification and conflict resolution of health care problems for older adults.

Examples of independent geriatric case management services include:

- Making multidimensional assessments of the older adult and primary caregiver at home or in the institutional setting for the purpose of providing information to plan short- and long-term goals.
- Providing information about care options in order to facilitate an appropriate plan of action that complements the older person's and family's needs and resources.
- Providing information as it relates to guardianship and competency issues.
- Arranging for appropriate care placement for the older person.
- Coordinating the continuum of community services and resources to enhance multidimensional functioning.
- Facilitating conflict resolution within the client system.
- Instituting a monthly support group for adult children of aging parents.

In terms of the selection and utilization of community resources, independent case managers have no vested interest in placing service providers, but rather select support agencies and personnel based on their ability to provide high-quality care and services that are cost-effective for both the older person and the family.

Independent geriatric case management services are designed for:

- Older persons who are struggling with life-style and health changes, but who do not qualify for Medicare-reimbursed home care services.
- Busy family members who have neither the time nor the experience to evaluate and monitor available resources.
- Adult children who live in a different city than their aging parents.
- Individuals without a health care background who are responsible for the health and well-being of older persons.

It is generally the primary caregiver of an older person who seeks the services of Community Care Consultants to coordinate care and resolve problems associated with chronic health care conditions. The target client group in an independent geriatric case management model are adult children of aging parents. Unlike most traditional health care delivery systems, Community Care Consultants provides case management services in the privacy of the older person's or family member's home or residence.

In the instance of long-term, long-distance caregiving for an elderly family member, the nurse case manager will assume 24-hour responsibility for all aspects of care for the older person. Verbal contracts are mutually established between the nurse case manager and the client system as to the problems, needs, and goals for nursing service.

There are a number of differences between independent geriatric case management services and traditional community-based nursing agencies that provide case management services.

One of the greatest differences between independent geriatric case management services and traditional nursing organizations is in the reimbursement mechanism. In independent geriatric case management, the older person and the family privately pay for the services of the case manager; in most traditional nursing agencies, reimbursement is primarily from third-party payers. Independent geriatric case management is not driven or circumscribed by third-party payers; therefore, nurse case managers are able to define and practice nursing without restrictions from regulatory agencies. This model works to the advantage of the independent nurse case manager in terms of greater time frames allotted in which to meet the needs of the client system. Clients are generally seen one or two times a week for several months.

In independent geriatric case management, it is the nurse who is responsible for executing the overall plan of care. The nurse has primary responsibility for collaborating with the various health care disciplines, and assumes responsibility for all aspects of health care coordination from a multidimensional perspective.

The independent geriatric case management model (see Figure 6) recognizes a "client system" for care coordination that includes the older adult, the family (generally, a primary caregiver), and the community. The nursing process of assessment, planning, implementation, and evaluation is applied to the entire "client system," rather

Figure 6
Independent Geriatric Case Management Model: Multidimensional Functional Approach

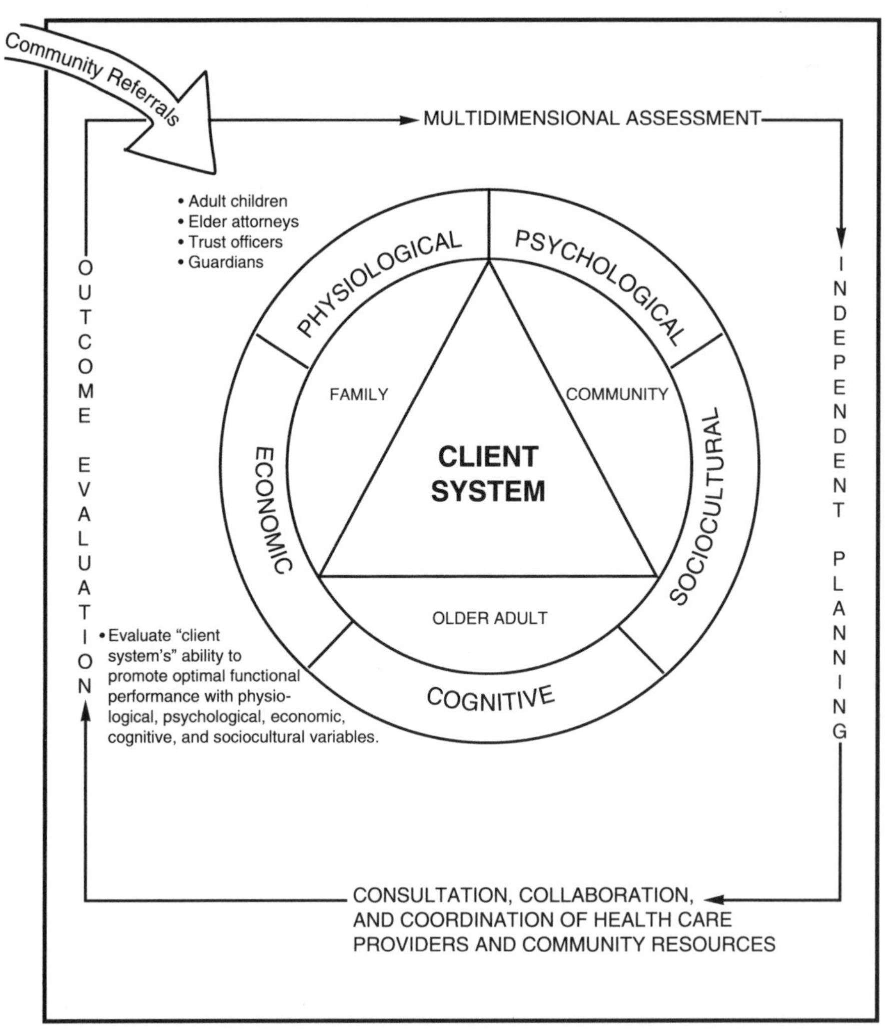

than to just the older person. The client system is viewed as a whole whose parts are in dynamic interaction, affected by physiological, psychological, sociocultural, cognitive, and economic variables.

Independent geriatric nurse case managers have been able to successfully demonstrate the following outcomes:

- Reducing unnecessary readmissions to the hospital.
- Postponing premature institutionalization.
- Promoting optimal family functioning.
- Enhancing and promoting the image of nursing in the community.
- Enhancing nursing autonomy, recruitment, and retention.

Because of the holistic nature of independent geriatric case management, nurses with advanced practice are best suited to provide comprehensive services to an older "client system."

Conclusion

Issues and Questions for the Future

Since case management by nurses has only recently become widespread, numerous questions about it have yet to be resolved. Zander, Etheredge, and Bower (1987), editors of *Nursing Case Management: Blueprints for Transformation,* raised the following significant questions concerning the future of case management by nurses:

- Does case management increase patients' levels of satisfaction with their care?
- Is there a significant difference in length of stay, resource utilization, and achievement of outcomes when case managers and non-case managers are compared?
- What is the most effective method of evaluating outcome achievement?
- Does the case management role increase the staff nurse's level of job satisfaction?
- What are the most effective and efficient ways of educating case managers for their role?
- What influence will case management have on curricula within nursing baccalaureate and master's programs?
- How does case management influence turnover, retention, and recruitment?
- Does case management fundamentally change the nursing image?
- What management styles and structures will be most effective with case managers?

As case management continues to evolve, additional questions and issues warrant future consideration:

- What is the most effective way to integrate the activities of case managers who interface with clients from various case management programs?
- Is there a need to refine the terminology of case management? It is possible that the nomenclature has not yet caught up with the current status of case management? To continue to refer to both "nurses in the case manager role" and "nursing case management" can cause confusion.
- In the future, will case managers be asked to serve more as cost-containment agents than is consistent with good case management? This could occur as managed care causes conflicting incentives for caregivers — both to care for patients' needs and to "look after" the financial interests of the delivery organization itself. What will be the effect of this potential conflict on outcomes of care and on nursing role satisfaction?
- What is the most effective method of drawing all disciplines into the case management process, without isolating or disenfranchising various disciplines or programs?
- What should be the relationship between nursing case management and the underlying nursing care delivery system within the organization? Additionally, which nursing care delivery system supports case management and assists in attaining the desired outcomes of case management programs?

Perhaps the most fundamental issue is raised by Maurin (1990) who, in her article "Case Management: Caring for Psychiatric Clients," asks, "What method of case management, delivered by whom, has what outcome for which patients?" This issue is likely to be discussed for years to come.

Appendix

Curriculum Outline on Nursing Assessment and Management of the Frail Elderly
(University of Kansas School of Nursing)*

Module 1 — Conceptual Framework for Comprehensive Functional Assessment and Management

- Introduction and self-care concepts
- The nursing process
- Standards of gerontological nursing practice
- Overview of case management
- The aging process: A review

Module 2 — Communication and Interviewing

- Interpersonal communication: A review
- Special concerns in communicating with the elderly
- The interviewing process

Module 3 — Comprehensive Functional Assessment

- Traditional versus standardized approaches to client assessment
- Purposes of standardized and comprehensive functional assessment

*This project was funded by the U.S. Department of Health and Human Services, Division of Nursing, through the Nursing Assessment and Management of the Frail Elderly (NAMFE) grant.

- Selection and examples of standardized assessment instruments
- Data collection
- Data analysis
- Nursing diagnosis

Module 4 — Assessment of the Informal Support System

- Overview of family caregiving
- Evaluating availability and capability of informal support system

Module 5 — Assessment of the Formal Support System

- The long-term care system
- Assessing community resources
- Developing a new community resource

Module 6 — Developing a Service Plan

- Introduction and prioritization of diagnoses
- Developing and refining the service plan
- Computerized service care planning

Module 7 — Implementation: Mobilizing the Informal and Formal Support Systems

- Strategies to mobilize family support system
- Interventions to build caregiving capacity
- Collaboration with the formal support system
- Advocacy for aged clients
- Case management/coordination of care

Module 8 — Evaluation: Outcomes of Care

- Introduction to evaluation of health care
- Conceptual and practical problems in evaluating care of the frail elderly
- Quality assurance from a systems perspective
- Measuring the impact of case management

References

American Nurses Association. 1974. *Standards of medical-surgical nursing practice.* Kansas City, Mo.: American Nurses Association.

______. 1980. *Nursing: A social policy statement.* Kansas City, Mo.: American Nurses Association.

______. 1982. *Standards of psychiatric and mental health nursing practice.* Kansas City, Mo.: American Nurses Association.

______. 1983. *Standards of maternal and child health nursing practice.* Kansas City, Mo.: American Nurses Association.

______. 1986a. *Standards of community health nursing practice.* Kansas City, Mo.: American Nurses Association.

______. 1986b. *Standards of home health nursing practice.* Kansas City, Mo.: American Nurses Association.

______. 1987a. *The scope of nursing practice.* Kansas City, Mo.: American Nurses Association.

______. 1987b. *Standards and scope of gerontological nursing practice.* Kansas City, Mo.: American Nurses Association.

______. 1987c. *Standards of practice for the primary health care nurse practitioner.* Kansas City, Mo.: American Nurses Association.

______. 1988. *Nursing case management.* Kansas City, Mo.: American Nurses Association.

______. 1991. *Standards of clinical nursing practice.* Kansas City, Mo.: American Nurses Association.

Bair, N.N.; Griswold, J.; and Head, J. 1989. Clinical RN involvement in bedside-centered case management. *Nursing Economic$* 7(3):C150-154.

Ballew, J.R. and Mink, G. 1986. *Case management in the human services.* Springfield, Ill.: Charles C. Thomas Publishers.

Caragno, G.; Applebaum, R.; Christianson, J.; Phillips, B.; Thornton, C.; and Will, J.1986. *The evaluation of the national long-term care demonstration: The planning and operational experience of the channeling projects,* volumes 1 and 2. Princeton, N.J.: Mathematica Policy Research, Inc.

Chapman, E. 1990. Nurse case management and hospital length of stay. Unpublished master's thesis. University of Arizona College of Nursing, Tucson.

Cohen, E.L. 1991. Nursing case management: Does it pay? *Journal of Nursing Administration* 21(4):20-25.

Dikmen, S. and Temkin, N. 1987. Determination of the effects of head injury and recovery in behavioral research. In *Neurobehavioral recovery from head injury,* eds. H.S. Levin, J. Grafman, and H.M. Eisenberg, pp. 73-87. New York: Oxford University Press.

Diller, L. and Ben-Yishay, Y. 1987. Outcomes and evidence in neuropsychological rehabilitation in closed head injury. In *Neurobehavioral recovery from head injury,* eds. H.S. Levin, J. Grafman, and H.M. Eisenberg, pp. 146-165. New York: Oxford University Press.

Ethridge, P. 1991. A nursing HMO: Carondelet St. Mary's experience. *Nursing Management* 22(7):22-27.

Ethridge, P. and Lamb, G. 1989. Professional nursing case management improves quality, access, and cost. *Nursing Management* 20(3):30-35.

Foster, J. and Hall, H. 1986. Public Health and AIDS. *Caring* 5(6):4-11, 73-78.

Genna, J. 1987. AIDS management. *Healthcare Forum Journal* (Nov./Dec.):18-48.

Grau, L. 1984. Case management and the nurse. *Geriatric Nursing* 5(8):372-375.

Joachim, G. 1989. The school nurse as case manager for chronically ill children. *Journal of School Health* 59(9):406-407.

Lamb, G. and Stempel, J. 1991. Nursing case management: The patient's experience. Presentation at the American Nurses Association Council of Nurse Researchers' International Nursing Research Conference, October 22-24, Los Angeles.

Maurin, J. 1990. Case management: Caring for psychiatric clients. *Journal of Psychosocial Nursing* 28(7):8-12.

Michaels, C. In press. Carondelet St. Mary's nursing enterprise. *Nursing Clinics of North America.*

Morrison, C. 1987. Establishing a therapeutic environment: Institutional resources. In *The person with AIDS: Nursing perspectives,* eds. J. Durham and F. Lashley-Cohen, pp. 110-125. New York: Springer.

Mundinger, M. 1984. Community-based care: Who will be the case managers? *Nursing Outlook* 32(6):294-295.

National Council on Aging. 1987. *Standards for case management.* Washington, D.C.: National Council on Aging.

New Jersey State Department of Health. 1983. Special child health services guidelines. Trenton, N.J.: New Jersey State Department of Health.

Nursing Assessment and Management of the Frail Elderly (NAMFE) Project. 1987. Curriculum of eight models on case management. NAMFE Project, Kansas City, Kan.

Nursing's agenda for health care reform. 1991. Kansas City, Mo.: American Nurses Publishing.

Orem, D. 1980. *Nursing concepts of practice.* New York: McGraw-Hill.

Pittman, D.C. 1989. Nursing case management: Holistic care for the deinstitutionalized chronically mentally ill. *Journal of Psychosocial Nursing* 27(11):23-27

Prime Health. 1987. Prime Health case management. Kansas City, Mo.: Prime Health.

Schwartz, S.; Goldman, H.; and Churgin, S. 1982. Case management for the chronic mentally ill: Models and dimensions. *Hospital and Community Psychiatry* 33(12):1006-1009.

Stanhope, M. and Lancaster, J. 1984. *Community health nursing: Process and practice for promoting health.* St. Louis: C.V. Mosby.

Zander, K. 1988a. Managed care within acute care settings: Design and implementation via nursing case management. *Health Care Supervisor* 6(2):27-43.

_____. 1988b. Nursing case management: Resolving the DRG paradox. *Nursing Clinics of North America* 23(3):503-520.

_____. 1988c. Nursing case management: Strategic management of cost and quality outcomes. *Journal of Nursing Administration* 18(5):23-30.

_____. 1990. Differentiating managed care and case management. *Definition* 5(2):1.

Zander, K.; Etheredge, M.; and Bower, K.; eds. 1987. *Nursing case management: Blueprints for transformation.* Boston: New England Medical Center Hospitals.

Bibliography

American Nurses Association. 1987. *Orthopaedic nursing practice: Process and outcome criteria for selected diagnoses*. Kansas City, Mo.: American Nurses Association.

Bachrach, L. 1989. Case management: Toward a shared definition. *Hospital and Community Psychiatry* 40(9):883-884.

Baier, M. 1987. Case management with the chronically mentally ill. *Journal of Psychosocial Nursing* 25(6):17-20.

Bennett, N. and Botti, J. 1989. New strategies for preterm labor. *American Journal of Primary Health Care* 14(4):27-28.

Blatter, C. 1989. Putting the TLC into LTC. *Best's Review* 90(8).

Borland, A.; McRae, J.; and Lycan, C. 1989. Outcomes of five years of continuous intensive case management. *Hospital and Community Psychiatry* 40(4):369-376.

Bremmer, A. 1989. A description of community health nursing practice with community-based elderly. *Community Health Nursing* 6(3):173-184.

Bricker, P. et al. 1988. Team approach enables frail elderly to stay home. *Health Progress* 60(6):46-49.

Bush, C.; Langford, M.; Rosen, P.; and Gott, W. 1990. Intensive case management for severely psychiatrically disabled adults. *Hospital and Community Psychiatry* 41(6):647-649.

Case management is just the ticket for home care. *Hospitals* 60(6).

Collins, L. 1989a. Case management reduces high-risk pregnancy cost. *Business Insurance* 23(8):70-73.

______. 1989b. Prenatal care gives birth to reduced costs. *Business Insurance* 23(8):69-72.

Combs, J. and Rusch, S. 1990. Creating a healing environment. *Health Progress* 73(4):38-41.

Cronin, C. and Makelbust, J. 1989. Case-managed care: Capitalizing on the CNS. *Nursing Management* 20(8):38-47.

Daniels, K. 1988. Will nurses control care at home? *Home Healthcare Nurse* 6(2):18-23.

Davidson, R.; Factor, R.; Gundlach, E.; and Adler, K. 1988. Psychiatric nursing roles in a community mental health center. *Community Mental Health Journal* 24(1):83-86.

Deitchman, W. 1980. How many case managers does it take to screw in a light bulb? *Hospital and Community Psychiatry* 5(8):788-789.

Downey-Dezell, A.; Comeau, E.; and Zander, K. 1988. Nursing case management: Managed care via the nursing case management model. In *Patients and purse-strings, volume II*, ed. J. Scherubel, pp. 253-264. New York: National League for Nursing.

Etheredge, M.L., ed. 1989. *Collaborative care: Nursing case management*. Chicago: American Hospital Association.

Ethridge, P. 1987. Building successful nursing care delivery systems for the future. Paper presented at the National Commission on Nursing Implementation Project Invitational Conference, November 4, San Diego, Calif.

Evashwick, C.; Ney, J.; and Siemon, J. 1985. *Case management: Issues for hospitals.* Chicago: American Hospital Association.

Fisher, K. 1987. QA update: Case management. *Quality Review Bulletin* 13(8):287-290.

Fondiller, S. 1991. How case management is changing the picture. *American Journal of Nursing* 91(1):62-80.

Forchuk, C.; Beaton, S.; Crawford, L.; Ide, L.; Voorberg, N.; and Bethune, J. 1989. Incorporating Peplau's theory and case management. *Journal of Psychosocial Nursing and Mental Health Services* 27(2):35-38.

Franklin, J.; Solovitz, B.; Mason, M.; Clemons, J.; and Miller, G. 1987. An evaluation of case management. *American Journal of Public Health* 77(6):674-678.

Freund, D. 1984. *Medicaid reform: Four studies of case management*. Washington, D.C.: American Enterprise Institute for Public Policy Research.

Goering, P.; Farkas, M.; Wasylenki, D.; Lancee, W.; and Ballantyne, R. 1988. Improved functioning for case management clients. *Psychosocial Rehabilitation Journal* 12(1):13-17.

Goering, P.; Wasylenki, D.; Farkas, M.; Lancee, W.; and Ballantyne, R. 1988. What difference does case management make? *Hospital and Community Psychiatry* 39(3):272-276.

Goldstrom, I. and Manderscheid, R. 1983. A descriptive analysis of community support program case managers serving the chronically mentally ill. *Community Mental Health* 19(1):17-26.

Green, G. 1984. Case management: State of the art. In *Coordinated Service Delivery Systems*, eds. R. Bennet, S. Frisch, B. Gurland, et al. New York: Haworth Press.

Guiliano, K. and Poirier, C. 1991. Nursing case management: Critical pathways to desirable outcomes. *Nursing Management* 22(3):52-57.

Harris, M. and Berman, H. 1986. Case management with the chronically mentally ill: A clinical perspective. *American Journal of Orthopsychiatry* 57(2):296-302.

Harrod, J. 1986. Defining case management in community support systems. *Psychosocial Rehabilitation Journal* 9(3):56-61.

Henderson, M. and Collard, A. 1988. Measuring quality in medical case management programs. *Quality Review Bulletin* 14(2):33-39.

Henderson, M.; Souder, B.; and Bergman, A. 1987. Measuring efficiencies of managed care. *Business and Health* 4(3):43-46.

Henderson, M. and Wallack, S. 1987. Evaluating case management for catastrophic illness. *Business and Health* 4(3):7-11.

Inglehart, J. 1983. Health policy report: Medicaid turns to prepaid managed care. *New England Journal of Medicine* 308(16):976-980.

Kanter, J. 1989. Clinical case management: Definition, principles, components. *Hospital and Community Psychiatry* 40(4):361-368.

Korenbot, C.; Showstack, J.; Loomis, A.; and Brandis, C. 1989. Birth weight outcomes in a teenage pregnancy case management project. *Journal of Adolescent Health Care* 10(2):97-104.

Kreiger, G. and Sullivan, J. 1987. The case for case management. *Occupational Health and Safety* 56(5):92.

Kurtz, L.; Badarozzi, D.; and Pollane, L. 1984. Case management in mental health. *Health and Social Work* 9(3):201-211.

Lamb, H. 1980. Therapist case managers: More than brokers of services. *Hospital and Community Psychiatry* 31(11):762-764.

LeClair, C. 1991. Introducing and accounting for RN case management. *Nursing Management* 22(3):44-51.

Long, T.; Katz, K.; and Pokorni, J. 1989. Developmental intervention with the chronically ill infant. *Infants and Young Children* 1(4):78-88.

Lulavage, A. 1991. RN-LPN teams: Toward unit nursing case management. *Nursing Management* 22(3):58-61.

Mazoway, J. 1987. Early intervention in high-cost care. *Business and Health* 4(3):12-16.

McKenzie, C.; Torkelson, N.; and Holt, M. 1989. Care and cost: Nursing case management improves both. *Nursing Management* 20(10):30-34.

Merrill, J.C. 1985. Defining case management. *Business and Health* 3(9):5-7.

Millenson, M. 1986. Managed care: Will it push providers against the wall? *Hospitals* 60(19):66-70.

Netting, F. and Williams, F. 1989. Ethical decision making in case management programs for the elderly. *Health Values* 13(3):3-8.

Newman, M.; Lamb, G.; and Michaels, C. In press. Nursing case management: The coming together of theory and practice. *Nursing and Health Care.*

Ogilvie, J.; Kirkwood, B.; Hay, L.; Sommers, L.; and Silverman, J. 1988. Moving toward collaborative practice on an orthopedic unit: Health care provider involvement in cost containment. *Orthopaedic Nursing* 7(6):35-39.

Parker, M. and Secord, L. 1988a. Case managers: Guiding the elderly through the health care maze. *American Journal of Nursing* 88(12):1674-1676.

______. 1988b. Private geriatric case management: Providers, services, and fees. *Nursing Economic$* 6(4):165-172.

Pierini, S. 1988. Case managing the elderly: Best bet for the future. *Health Progress* 69(11):42-45.

Plum, K. 1989. Analysis of a capitation plan for the chronically mentally ill. *Nursing Economic$* 7(5):250-256.

Possin, B. 1991. A consortium introduces RN case management regionwide. *Nursing Management* 22(3):62-64.

Rapp, C. and Wintersteen, R. 1989. The strengths model of case management: Results from twelve demonstrations. *Psychosocial Rehabilitation Journal* 13(1):23-32.

Reinhard, S. 1988. Case managing community services for hip-fractured elders. *Orthopaedic Nursing* 7(5):42-49.

Rogers, M.; Riordan, J.; and Swindle, D. 1991. Community-based nursing case management pays off. *Nursing Management* 22(3):30-38.

Rusch, S. 1986. Continuity of care: From hospital unit into home. *Nursing Management* 17(12):31-41.

Salmon, M. and Peoples-Sheps, M. 1989. Infant mortality and public health nursing. *Nursing Outlook* 37(1):6-7.

Salmond, S. 1990. In-hospital case management: Responses to common questions and concerns. *Orthopaedic Nursing* 9(1):38-40.

Sinnen, M. and Schifalacqua, M. 1991. Coordinated care in a community hospital. *Nursing Management* 22(3):38-43.

Smith, S.S. 1985. Traumatic head injuries. In *Neurological rehabilitation,* ed. D.A. Umphred, pp. 249-288. St. Louis: C.V. Mosby.

Steinberg, R. and Carter, G. 1982. *Case management and the elderly: A handbook for planning and administering programs.* Lexington, Mass.: Lexington Books.

______. 1983. *Case management and the elderly.* Lexington, Mass.: D.C. Health & Co.

Wagner, D. 1987. Client care management. *Caring* 6(12):12-14.

Wahlstedt, P. and Blaser, W. 1986. Nurse case management for the frail elderly: A curriculum to prepare nurses for that role. *Home Healthcare Nurse* 4(2):30-35.

Whitman, M. 1991. Case management in head injury rehabilitation. *Rehabilitation Nursing* 16(1):19-22.

Wimberly, E. and Blazye, S. 1989. Monitoring patient outcomes following discharge: A computerized geriatric case management system. *Health and Social Work* 14(4):269-276.

Worley, N.; Drago, L.; and Hadley T. 1990. Improving the physical health-mental interface for the chronically and mentally ill: Could nurse case managers make a difference? *Archives of Psychiatric Nursing* 4(2):8-13.

Zander, K. 1990. The 1990s: Core values, core change. *Frontiers in Health Services Management* 7(2):28-32.

_____. 1991. Case management in acute care: Making the connections. *The Case Manager* 2(1):39-43.

Zitter, M. 1989. Don't shy from seniors: They're your future. *Modern Health Care* 19(12):36.